# DES:
## The Complete Story

# DES:
## The Complete Story

## by Cynthia Laitman Orenberg

Introduction by Howard Ulfelder, M.D.

ST. MARTIN'S PRESS
• NEW YORK

Library of Congress Cataloging in Publication Data

Orenberg, Cynthia.
    DES, the complete story.

    Bibliography: p.
    1. Diethylstilbestrol—Toxicology.    2. Diethylstilbestrol—Side effects.
    3. Fetus—Effect of drugs on.    4. Vagina—Cancer.    5. Generative or-
gans—Abnormalities.    I. Title.
RA1242.D48074          363.1'94          81-13607
ISBN 0-312-18081-0                        AACR2

Illustrated by Joan Kozel
Design by Laura Hammond
10  9  8  7  6  5  4  3

For Kate
and
for all DES daughters, sons
and mothers

"Ulysses, it is said, went off to fight the Trojan War. Battle completed, he attempted to return home but found it necessary to pass through a series of often unpleasant adventures over 20 years, to arrive once again at his starting point. The Ulysses syndrome in medicine consists of a series of adverse events stemming from a procedure or a therapy that should never have been undertaken, sometimes requiring heroic measures just to get back to the starting point."

James F. Fries, M.D., Associate Professor of Medicine, Stanford University Medical School. *From* "The Approach to the Rheumatic Disease Patient," published in *Comprehensive Therapy*, August 1979.

# Table of Contents

# Acknowledgments

I could not have written this book without the encouragement, help, and cooperation of many people.

First, I wish to express my profound gratitude to the officers and members of DES Action, Inc., who gave me their unstinting cooperation, supplied me with information, and shared with me their personal experiences. I especially wish to thank Nancy Adess, president; Dolores Wallgren, vice-president; Libby Saks, secretary; Pat Cody, treasurer; and Susan White, editor of the DES Action *Voice*. These people also reviewed chapters 4 and 6 and made many valuable suggestions. I also wish to thank Marilyn Butler who sent me much useful information, and Evelyn Goldberg and Faye Cohen.

Hannah Cook-Wallace and Andrea Goldstein generously allowed me to recount their personal experiences and for that, I am in their debt.

My deep appreciation to the following physicians who, by allowing me to interview them, contributed their time and expertise to this book. They are, in alphabetical order, Dr. Richard Dowden, Department of Surgery, Cleveland Clinic; Dr. Philip Farrell, professor of pediatrics, University of Wisconsin Medical School; Dr. William Gill, Department of Urology, University of Chicago Pritzker School of Medicine; Dr. E. Robert Greenberg, Dartmouth Medical School; Dr. Leonard Kurland, chairman of the Department of Epidemiology and Medical Statistics, Mayo Clinic; Dr. Raul Matallana, associate professor of radiology, University of Wisconsin Medical School; Dr. Ben Peckham, chairman of the Department of Obstetrics and Gynecology, University of Wisconsin Medical School; Dr. David Rose, professor of oncology and human nutrition, University of Wisconsin Medical School; Dr. Adolf Stafl, professor of obstetrics and gynecology, Medical College of Wisconsin (Milwaukee); Dr. Morton Stenchever, chairman of the Department of Obstetrics and Gynecology, University of Washington (Seattle); and Dr. David Uehling, professor of urology, University of Wisconsin Medical School. I especially wish to thank Dr. David Rose, who reviewed chapter 2 and Dr. William Gill, who reviewed chapter 5.

My deep appreciation to Stephan Beyer, who not only reviewed chapter 8 on DES and the law for correctness, but also helped me to understand some basic legal theories. My sincere gratitude, too, to Allan Ashman, executive director of the National Conference of Bar Examiners, and Dr. Richard Moll, professor of engineering, University of Wisconsin, for sending me valuable material relevant to chapter 8.

I wish to thank Mr. Daniel Griffen, executive director of the Iowa State University Research Foundation, who graciously sent me information about the work of Dr. Wise Burroughs.

Ms. Joan Kozel, medical illustrator at the University of Wisconsin Medical School, deserves special recognition for her skilled drawings which illumine the texts of chapters 2, 4, and 5.

My fond appreciation to two friends and fellow writers, Judy Kesselman and Franklynn Peterson, who helped me to take this book from an idea to a reality. And my appreciation to the two people who first suggested I write this book, Dr. Tim and Mrs. Rita Harrington.

I also wish to thank my first editor at St. Martin's, Rebecca Martin, and my second editor, Marcia Markland, and my agent, Amy Berkower, whose incisive comments and constant encouragement helped me to turn this book into a finished manuscript.

If this book is of value, it is due to the help of these people; what mistakes you find are mine alone.

This litany of thanks would not be complete without acknowledging my husband, Alan, and my daughters, Kate and Rachel, who cheerfully tolerated my year-long preoccupation with this book and whose confidence and whose love never flagged.

Cynthia Laitman Orenberg

# Introduction

It is just ten years since the stilbestrol story first came to public notice. By its uniqueness and implications it inevitably evoked rapid and widespread responses. Much already has been written in professional journals, and a considerable amount also in the newspapers, magazines, and books read by the public at large. Cynthia Laitman Orenberg's book is none the less welcome, for it combines, in eminently readable prose, the autobiographical view of one who is personally deeply involved and the scientific facts which one must understand in order to comprehend how and why the stilbestrol disorders evolved and what the lessons are for each of us.

In other words, it tells, as it claims to do, the complete story, often balancing personal and anecdotal observations with descriptive and explanatory data in the best tradition of science writing for the laity. From time to time we glimpse more than a hint of criticism of doctors and of drug manufacturers, but surely knowing the circumstances this can be understood. No important feature of the subject has been neglected. The situation as it stands for DES daughters, DES mothers, and DES sons is thoroughly dealt with and even the DES fathers, an overlooked but significantly affected group, come in for a modicum of attention when the emotional aspects are reviewed.

It has given me great satisfaction to study and preface this manuscript, because I have lived longer than any other human being with the knowledge that stilbestrol carried the potential for harm. I know this because I was the doctor asked by the concerned mother who first raised the possibility [that DES might have caused her daughter's cancer]. And although my reply at the time was in the negative, my instinct told me forthwith that it might just possibly be so and, if it proved to be true, what calamities might yet be in store. As the weight of evidence accumulated and it became even more certain that DES was the culprit, I was brought face to face with the necessity to report the findings scientifically and at the same time to inform the public at large. Doing this was made no easier by the fact that I knew and respected many of the physicians who had published on the subject. Indeed, I had studied under them. On the other hand, it was clearly imperative that the practice of prescribing DES in pregnancy should end at once, and desirable that the message should be delivered in a manner least likely to create emotional disturbance in the individuals who had already been exposed.

*DES—The Complete Story* is very much in this tradition. The facts are clearly displayed, but there is careful emphasis directed to those which are a source of emotional support, such as the extremely low incidence of adenocarcinoma in girls, the high probability of successful child-bearing in the DES daughters, and the ease of correction of anatomic anomalies in both daughters and sons.

Doubtless, much remains to be learned from this experience and from the clinical and basic research that it has stimulated. Ten years is a very short time for the development of a body of new knowledge. This book, at this moment, offers the interested lay reader a clear picture of the stilbestrol disorders, and a point of reference for whatever the future still has to tell us.

*Howard Ulfelder, M.D.*
April 1981

# Prologue

Take a brand new drug. Then, based mostly on theory, manufacture that drug and prescribe it in huge quantities to millions of patients. Don't stop for more than 30 years, even though the drug is proven ineffective, until it's shown—beyond doubt—to cause cancer.

What have you got? You've got a medical fiasco. You've got the story of DES, short for *di*ethyl*s*tilbestrol. DES, an artificial estrogen, was given to pregnant women in the belief that it would prevent miscarriage. Instead, it caused cancer in some of the children born of these pregnancies, and benign abnormalities in most of them.

The DES story is my story, too. And my daughter's. And that of the three million other mothers who were given DES, and their children. The story needs telling for all of us because we need to know how to live with what the drug has done to us. But it also needs telling for everyone else who uses the services of physicians because the fiasco could happen again in other ways and with other "medical miracles."

What happened with DES is only one example of the consequences of thinking that modern medicine is infallible, that the physician is sacrosanct, and that the patient (particularly the *woman* patient) is an object to be "done to."

Although the infallibility of modern medicine is challenged and belied continually by a steady stream of newer and "even better" treatments, and although laws and codes of professional ethics abound to regulate the activities of physicians, patients themselves too often remain *shlubs** when it comes to their own health care.

This book is written to document the DES story, a shameful but illustrative episode in the maturation of the medical profession. And, it is written to help those affected by DES to

---

*Shlub*—A jerk; a foolish, stupid, or unknowing person. Fred Kogos, *A Dictionary of Yiddish Slang and Idioms.*

cope with the consequences by offering practical and realistic advice.

But the book is also written to help *all* health care consumers overcome the ineptness, the ignorance, and the paralyzing awe of doctors that have characterized too many patients for too long, and that have made them vulnerable.

*Cynthia Laitman Orenberg*
Madison, Wisconsin

# 1 · My Doctor Prescribes DES: Pregnancy Insurance

In spite of my dislike of drugs, in spite of my science background, in spite of my determination to do everything "right" during my pregnancy, I am a statistic in the DES story. And so, of course, is my daughter.

For me, it began when I became pregnant with Kate. Alan and I had been married three years before, when I was 27 years old. Both of us wanted children very much.

I had graduated from college six years earlier and—with my degree in biology—had worked full-time as a medical research assistant. My first job was at the Sloan-Kettering Institute for Cancer Research in New York. Although I worked with cancer (albeit in rats and mice) every day, I had little sensitivity to cancer as a deadly human disease from which people suffered and often died.

In 1962 I left Sloan-Kettering and my parents' home and moved to Boston. I had rented a tiny, furnished apartment three blocks from Harvard Square in Cambridge. The Boston strangler still had eight victims to go when I moved, and my parents nervously telephoned almost daily to assure themselves of my safety.

Still, life was lovely. In addition to thoroughly enjoying the heady feeling of being on my own, I had been very fortunate to find a job I loved. I had become the research assistant to Dr. K. Frank Austen, a doctor who was just starting his laboratory at the Massachusetts General Hospital in Boston, one of the best hospitals in the country. Dr. Austen was intense and dedicated, I was his doggedly faithful assistant, and in time his laboratory produced advancements in immunology that have earned him world renown as an immunologist.

It was during my third year in Dr. Austen's employ that I was introduced to my future husband. Five months later, Alan and I were married. I resigned from my job with Dr. Austen, gave up an opportunity to go to graduate school, and settled down to have babies. I had been raised to think that working was something a woman did to pass time until she could marry and have a family.

When I became pregnant two years later, Alan and I were delighted. We were moving from an apartment to our first home and I drove myself to scrub floors, paint walls, and hang curtains. One day, when Alan was out of town on business, I became aware of a cramping sensation barely rippling through my pelvis. I tried to ignore it, but just a few hours later, I started spotting blood. I called my obstetrician, who had me come in for an examination, gave me an injection of progesterone (one of the two major female hormones; *see* chapter 2, page 15), and sent me home with instructions to go to bed.

In spite of this treatment, by evening the ripple of cramps had turned into grinding shockwaves of pain. At midnight, the legendary "dark hour," I miscarried. I was just beginning my fourth month of pregnancy.

The miscarriage left me with a profound sense of loss. When I conceived again eight months later I was ecstatic and vowed to myself that I would do everything right for this pregnancy. I even gave up cigarette smoking, although I had been a pack-a-day smoker for seven years. But, in spite of my plenty-of-rest, all-the-right-foods regimen, I started spotting again in my second month.

This time, my doctor became quite concerned and said we

could take no chances. He told me that since I had miscarried and was threatening to do so again, it could mean my body was not producing enough of its own female hormones to sustain pregnancy. He said that the way to prevent another miscarriage was for me to take hormones.

The suggestion that I take drugs made me feel uneasy. Although I didn't know a great deal about hormones, I knew enough to understand that they had wide-ranging effects on the body. I knew, for example, that cortisone given to arthritis sufferers works to reduce inflammation and so to ease the pain, but it also causes a bloated, typically "moon-faced" appearance in patients who take it for any length of time. I knew, too, from my years working for Dr. Austen that hormones are also given to kidney transplant patients to suppress their natural immune systems so the transplanted kidneys won't be rejected. And, I knew that because these hormones suppressed the patients' own natural defenses against germs, they were unable to fight even common bacteria and viruses and often died of simple infections. Although these immuno-suppressive hormones were not the "female" hormones my obstetrician was proposing to give to me, they were, nevertheless, related chemicals, and my apprehensions grew.

Besides being apprehensive of hormones, I was fearful of any drugs during pregnancy. By then, 1968, there was evidence that certain drugs (including the chemicals in cigarettes) taken by pregnant women could damage an unborn child. Only a few years earlier, the thalidomide tragedy had attracted our horrified attention as pictures of limbless children—victims of prenatal exposure to thalidomide—made the front pages of newspapers across the country.

"Could these hormones hurt my baby?" I asked my doctor. "No, no," he assured me, "pregnant women have been taking them for at least 20 years and, believe me, nothing happens to them or their babies."

I keenly wanted to bear a child, and so I put my trust in the doctor. After all, I told myself, he was the one with the medical education. If he said it was safe, and it could help my pregnancy, who was I to argue?

So we started the hormone treatments and in my sixth week of pregnancy I became a DES mother. I started with 5 milligrams daily and each two weeks thereafter; on doctor's orders I increased this amount by 5 more milligrams until by the middle of my eighth month, I was taking 125 milligrams daily. To give you an idea of how large a dose this is, a daily dose of many of today's birth control pills contains no more than *half a milligram* of estrogen; the "morning-after" birth control pill calls for 50 milligrams daily of DES, and the effective dose of DES for prostate cancer treatment is 2 to 5 milligrams daily. In other words, *each day I was taking the equivalent amount of estrogen contained in up to nine months' worth of birth control pills.*

In addition to these daily doses of DES, my doctor prescribed a "little extra insurance" for me in the form of progesterone injections. I got one injection each week, alternating in each hip. The injections hurt and after several weeks, I developed painful lumps at the injection sites. When my hips broke out in itchy, red welts and there was no clear spot to insert the hypodermic needle, the doctor suggested I switch to Enovid™, a birth *control* pill, which contained artificial progesterone and an artificial estrogen. I was to take Enovid *in addition to* DES, throughout my pregnancy.

Along with all these hormones, my doctor also prescribed three weeks of bed rest. With the 20/20 wisdom of hindsight, we know now that it was the bed rest alone, if it was *anything* I consciously did, that helped preserve my pregnancy.

Once I got through my fourth month, my pregnancy proceeded without incident, and on May 1, 1969, I gave birth to Kate. She was healthy and beautiful. I forgot about the DES I had taken, and absorbed myself in motherhood. That is, until Kate was two years old.

We were living in Framingham, Massachusetts, a town about 20 miles west of Boston, and I was a full-time housewife and mother. It was the spring of 1971. I had just finished my morning chores and had poured myself a second cup of coffee. That morning's Boston *Globe* was spread on the kitchen table before me. Kate was presiding happily over a tattered menagerie of stuffed animals under a quilting of warm, morning sun coming through the big front window. I looked back at my newspaper and as I scanned the front page, my eyes came to rest on a small story—just a few paragraphs—but it jolted me like an earthquake. It told of an article in that week's issue of the prestigious *New England Journal of Medicine,* which reported a connection between a rare form of vaginal cancer in young girls and an artificial estrogen their mothers had taken during pregnancy. The artificial estrogen, the article went on, was diethylstilbestrol—DES for short—and the women were given it to prevent miscarriage.

The warm and cozy feeling of the morning vanished. I thought of all those little white pills of DES I had swallowed, and I wanted to vomit.

I suddenly felt frozen and started to shudder uncontrollably. How could this terrible thing happen to my baby? Why had I ever agreed to take DES? Why hadn't I followed my instincts? The self-recriminations were terrible, but not nearly as bad as the terror that my baby might get cancer, that she might suffer and die because I hadn't listened to my inner voice which told me drugs were bad.

I wanted to talk with someone, but Alan, again, was out of town on business. And if I called my mother, she'd worry even more than I. I pulled myself together and decided the logical person to talk with was my doctor. When I arrived at his office, he was his usual pleasant self. Afraid to offend him, I timidly ventured a question about DES and cancer. His response was swift and superficial. "Don't worry," he said, "that cancer is so rare. Just forget about it." But of course I couldn't forget about it, although at the time, there seemed nothing more I could do.

I did not see any more articles on DES and further, I did not seem to have the energy—physical or intellectual—to pursue it. Ever since Kate's birth, I felt consumed with fatigue.

"Bone-tired," the expression is. But I felt that way all the time. At first, I attributed it to Kate's nighttime feedings. Not being able to sleep more than three or four consecutive hours at a time, night after night, exacts a price, but the price I was paying seemed excessive. Although Kate had long since outgrown her need for a nighttime feeding, my tiredness never went away. In fact, it seemed to get worse. When my hair, which I had always been proud of, lost its shine and started falling out, my obstetrician in Boston had chalked it up to "postpartum syndrome," symptoms many women have following the delivery of their babies. For the same reason, he told me not to worry about my swollen fingers and legs. "Wear elastic stockings," he advised. "Remember, you're a mother now." Was motherhood really supposed to do such wretched things to a woman? Why, when I looked into the mirror, didn't I see some beatific madonna instead of a baggy-eyed, sallow-faced caricature of myself?

I began to realize that my vision and hearing, as well as my appearance, had begun to fade. I decided that perhaps another doctor might help me, but I was wrong. The second doctor I went to, an internist in Framingham, told me I was suffering from "housewife's syndrome," a neurotic reaction. He never even took a blood test! I, dizzy with exhaustion, believed him. I had never had a psychosomatic symptom in my whole life, but I was too tired and too timid to protest.

By the time we moved to Madison, Wisconsin, the following spring, just before Kate's third birthday, my right foot had grown numb. During a visit to my daughter's new pediatrician, I casually mentioned that I had had no feeling in one of my feet for three weeks. I must have been feeling particularly poorly that day to have said anything at all, because I fully expected him to label me a hypochondriac, as the other doctors had. Instead, he asked me to take off my shoe. He then poked my foot with the end of a paper clip, and when he realized I could feel nothing, he made an appointment for me to see an internist. I was to see the doctor in a few days.

When the morning of my appointment arrived, I allowed myself an extra hour to dress and make up. It had been so long since I had felt pretty, and since I was about to be scrutinized closely, I invested what for me at that time was a herculean effort in my appearance.

When I walked into the doctor's office, and he took his first look at me, his eyes widened. "Do you always look this way?" he asked.

"Why, no," I replied with a maidenly blush. "I spent some extra time today...."

"I'm sorry," he apologized. "I don't mean that you look good. You're jaundiced, your eye is nearly swollen shut, you're edematous, and you're covered with black-and-blue marks."

"You mean," I asked incredulously, "there's something wrong with me?"

"I'm afraid so," he answered.

And I, after three years of feeling increasingly ill but believing those who had told me I was imagining things, could only feel relief at this new doctor's conclusion. Now, maybe, they could do something to make me feel better.

The results of many blood tests showed that I was severely hypothyroid—that my thyroid gland had ceased to function—and that I was suffering from acute anemia. Had I gone on without medical attention, I would have been dead by now. With the daily thyroid supplements I have taken ever since, I feel fine.

I mention this illness because I believe it was induced by the large quantities of DES I took during pregnancy (*see* chapter 2; section on thyroid, page 19). I describe the desultory medical attention I received at the beginning because it illustrates another problem—namely, that too many male physicians automatically assume a woman's medical complaints to be symptoms of neurotic behavior. (I will discuss medical sexism at greater length in chapter 10.)

Once I started thyroid therapy and I was feeling well again,

I noticed that more articles had begun to appear in newspapers and magazines about DES. Unfortunately, many were little more than lurid reminders of the worst effects of DES, including bone-chilling descriptions of teenaged girls screaming in pain and dying of their DES-induced cancers.

What the media played up, the doctors tended to play down. Those I spoke with still insisted that there was little need to worry. By that time, I knew that there were many thousands of women like myself who, perhaps, knew even less about DES than I did. During the following years, I began keeping a file on every piece of information on DES that I could find. When I went to work as a medical editor at the University of Wisconsin Medical School, I started collecting in earnest. Armed with my experience as a medical writer and editor, and with access to the medical library, my single folder soon swelled to fill an entire drawer in a file cabinet.

People at the university who knew of my interest soon started calling me for information, and acquaintances at the local Cancer Information Service began using me as a resource person for DES information.

The more I talked about DES and the more I learned, the more in control I felt of my own fears. Still, I worried about how I was going to tell Kate about the whole business—about how I, her mother who loves her so much, had taken a drug that could cause serious problems for her.

The problem of how to break the news to Kate was solved for me. I was driving Kate and our younger daughter, Rachel, to school one morning when a prerecorded interview I had done for a state-wide radio station came on.

The interview I had given was completely candid—a 15-minute precis of my experience with DES, the drug's risks, and my own fears and responses. Kate's reaction to the interview was surprisingly matter-of-fact.

"As long as I'm stuck with it," she said, "at least I have a mom who knows about it."

During this last year, as I have worked on this book, Kate's attitude has remained basically the same. Although she has since learned of the probability that she will have DES-related *benign* abnormalities, she takes it all in stride.

Alan was skeptical when Kate, then 11 years old, wanted to watch a dramatization about DES on a recent television show. "Don't worry, Dad," she said, "I already know the worst that can happen." She watched the show with interest and, true to her own reassurances, no trace of anxiety.

So far, so good. But, of course, Kate is still very young, one of the youngest of all DES daughters, and we still won't know for several years how the DES I took will affect Kate. But her calm attitude makes dealing with the matter much easier. She knows that soon after she gets her first period, she will start her DES examinations every six months, and continue them indefinitely.

Were it not for my DES experience, I would feel quite removed from the thousands, perhaps millions, of other victims of scientifically created fiascos—soldiers with permanent nerve disorders because they were exposed to the highly toxic defoliant, Agent Orange, or the leukemia victims of today who were the nuclear blast witnesses of three or more decades ago, or the Japanese children who lie helplessly spastic and profoundly retarded because their mothers ate fish polluted with mercury from industrial wastes, or the thalidomide babies of the sixties who were born without arms and legs because their mothers were given the tranquilizer to combat the nausea of early pregnancy. The list could go on.

If you are like me, when you hear stories like these, like the DES fiasco, you say to yourself, "Thank God, it's not me," and you go on your way. But there is a good reason for you to pay more attention, to become more aware, and to learn to protect yourself.

Because you—like me—are vulnerable. If you are not informed, if you are not aware, believe me. It can happen to you.

# 2·DES—What, Where, Why, When, Who, and How

*"[Hormones] conduct the whole performance; they are like the master switch that awakens a city to activity, or the throttle that controls an engine, or the red cape that excites the bull."*

ISAAC ASIMOV,
*The Intelligent Man's Guide to Science*

Some years ago, the actor Tony Curtis starred in a movie about a man who had become known as The Great Imposter. In real life, the man—Fred Demara—had gotten along for nearly 20 years by successfully (and fraudulently) impersonating other people.

Although he had little formal education, Demara had convincingly played many roles, among them a monk, a high-ranking naval officer, and a physician. So skillful was Demara at simulating a professional demeanor that even after he was caught and arrested, his "patients" swore that he was a great doctor!

Like Fred Demara, DES is a great imposter. DES acts like the natural hormone, estrogen, but underneath the "act," it is definitely something else. Chemically and in some important biological ways, DES is very different from natural estrogen.

Estrogen and other naturally occurring hormones are steroids. All steroid substances, including the male and female hormones, cholesterol, and cortisone have a chemically distinct, four-ring structure. (*See* illustration.) DES, an artificial compound concocted in the laboratory, does not have this distinctive make-up. In short, it is a "ringer."

Not being a steroid, DES is *fundamentally different* from the

Progesterone    Testosterone    Cholesterol

Estradiol (estrogen)    Cortisone    Diethylstibestrol

natural sex hormones, including estrogen, in spite of the fact that it behaves empirically like estrogen. Enigmatically, the doctors who for so many years prescribed DES seemed never to wonder that perhaps this fundamental chemical difference might result in fundamentally different biological effects, some of which are discussed later in this chapter.

Just as puzzling, DES-prescribing physicians never thought that they might be tampering dangerously with nature. Ironically, DES itself was a product of a tremendous boom in knowledge about hormones—about their immense biological powers and about the fine-tuning of the human endocrine hormone system. Yet, despite the fact that doctors were feeding women huge overloads of a hormonally active chemical, the advocates of DES never seemed to worry about unbalancing these hormonal powers or upsetting that fine tuning.

These oversights are all the more difficult to understand in light of how the endocrine glands work. In order to appreciate the potency and delicate balance of our hormone systems, and how DES can adversely affect the human body, it is necessary to understand the workings of some important endocrine glands.

# • ABOUT HORMONES IN GENERAL

Hormones, named after a Greek word meaning "to rouse to activity," are the chemical spark plugs of our bodies. They are secreted by an amazingly diverse lot of structures called glands, and perform a vast array of biological jobs without which life would be impossible.

There are basically two types of glands, the exocrine and the endocrine. The main difference between the two is that the exocrine—which include the salivary, sweat, digestive, and mammaries—release their secretions through small tubules or ducts. The endocrine glands are ductless, and their secretions are absorbed directly into the bloodstream.

The endocrine glands include the ovaries, testicles, adrenals, pancreas, thyroid, parathyroids, thymus, and pituitary. (*See* illustration.) Collectively, these glands are responsible for the growth and development of every cell in our bodies, the development and maintenance of our sexual characteristics, our ability to digest food, the correct balance of fluids and electrolytes (sodium, potassium, and calcium), and the regulation of our blood pressure.

All the endocrine glands function and interact in delicate harmony. If one gland should over- or underproduce a particular hormone, this will cause a compensating reaction in the rest of the system, more often than not resulting in ill health. While the following information may seem a bit technical, I offer it as a basis for better understanding the development of DES as an antiabortive agent.

## The Pituitary Gland

The pituitary gland is indeed "the switch that awakens a city to activity." It is the central control for the endocrine system—the "master gland." This tiny lobe- and stalk-shaped bit of tissue is nestled protectively in about the center of the skull, just under the front portion of the brain and behind the nose.

# ENDOCRINE GLANDS

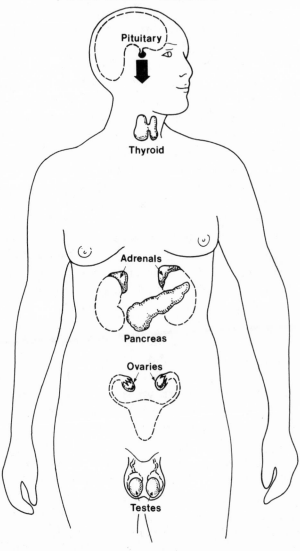

The front lobe of the pituitary produces at least six major hormones, which, in turn, stimulate all the other endocrine glands to action. These six hormones are (1) growth hormone, (2) thyrotropic hormone, (3) adrenocorticotrophic hormone, (4) follicle-stimulating hormone, (5) luteinizing hormone, and (6) luteotrophic hormone.

*Growth hormone.* This is secreted in large quantities from before birth through adolescence, and stimulates the growth of virtually every cell in the body.

Once adulthood is reached, the pituitary gland responds to some unknown signal and drastically reduces the secretion of growth hormone. An undersecretion in childhood causes dwarfism; an oversecretion can cause the unabated growth leading to giantism (hence, the term "pituitary giant").

If the pituitary malfunctions in adulthood by resuming a large production of growth hormone, a condition known as acromegaly results. The soft bone, or cartilage, is mainly affected so that the nose, forehead, jaw, hands, and feet are spurred to exaggerated, sometimes monstrous, overgrowth. Old movie buffs may remember the acromegalic actor who put his pituitary disorder to work by playing a villain called "The Creeper."

*Thyrotropic hormone.* This pituitary hormone stimulates the thyroid gland to secrete and release into the bloodstream thyroid hormone. Too much thyrotropic hormone produces Graves's disease, or hyperthyroidism, in which the thyroid gland overproduces, resulting in a rapid heart rate, increased metabolic activity, unusual nervousness, fatigue, insomnia, and bulging eyes. Too little thyrotropic hormone, and the thyroid gland slows down or stops its functioning.

*Adrenocorticotrophic hormone.* This hormone, known for short as ACTH, regulates the secretions of the outer shell of the adrenal glands. These secretions are the corticosteroids of which cortisone is perhaps the most popularly known.

As with thyrotropic hormone, too much or too little ACTH produces a parallel increase or decrease in the activity of its target gland.

The following three hormones are known collectively as the gonadotropic hormones, and are secreted in vastly increased quantities as a child approaches puberty. Through their influence on the sex organs (or gonads), the gonadotropic hormones effectively regulate and control sexual maturation.

*Follicle-stimulating hormone.* In the female, the follicle-stimulating hormone (FSH) spurs the development of the cells (or follicles) surrounding each egg (ovum) in the ovaries.

In the male, FSH promotes the development of the seminiferous tubules, that part of the testes which produces sperm.

*Luteinizing hormone.* The production of testosterone as a boy reaches puberty is directly dependent on the amount of luteinizing hormone produced by the pituitary.

In the female, the combination of luteinizing hormone and follicle-stimulating hormone causes the ovaries to secrete estrogens. The cyclic production of luteinizing hormone during the middle of each monthly menstrual cycle also causes ovulation.

*Luteotrophic hormone.* Following ovulation, the follicle that has just released the mature ovum turns into a small, hormone-producing organ in its own right called the corpus luteum (from the Latin meaning "yellow body"). Under the influence of luteotrophic hormone, the corpus luteum produces large quantities of estrogen and progesterone, which prepare a woman's body each month for possible pregnancy.


## Ovaries

In the nonpregnant, mature female, the ovaries are the major producers of estrogen and progesterone, the female sex hormones. During pregnancy, the placenta secretes large quantities of both hormones as well. (Following menopause, the ovaries greatly slow down production of both hormones.)

*Estrogen.* There are three components of estrogen—estradiol, estrone, and estriol. For the sake of convenience, I will use the single, collective term, estrogen.

Physiology books describe the basic function of estrogen as causing cellular proliferation, especially in those parts of the body involved in reproduction.

Before puberty, estrogen is secreted in only small quantities. As puberty is reached, the pituitary stimulates a greatly increased production of estrogen, causing the uterus, fallopian tubes, and vagina to enlarge and mature.

Estrogen causes an increase in the size of the vaginal labia and the development of milk ducts in the breasts, as well as the generalized growth of the breasts. Under the influence of estrogen, bones grow, the pelvis broadens, skin and hair remain soft (as opposed to a toughening process in males), and the kidneys resorb greater amounts of calcium, phosphorus, chloride, and water.

As a woman ages and enters menopause, the natural decline in production of estrogen can produce "hot flashes," irritability, fatigue, anxiety, and osteoporosis (loss of calcium from the bones).

In about 15 percent of women, these symptoms are severe enough to induce them to seek medical help, and it has been a common practice during the last 40 years to administer estrogen—often DES—to temporarily relieve these symptoms of menopause. The consequences of this treatment will be discussed elsewhere in this book.

*Progesterone.* Unlike estrogen, which has a generalized effect on the entire body, progesterone functions to prepare and maintain a woman's body for pregnancy. It is secreted during the last half of the menstrual cycle by the corpus luteum, and by the placenta during pregnancy. It prepares the uterus for implantation of the fertilized ovum, and the breasts for lactation.

## Placenta

The placenta is a roundish body of tissue attached like an upside-down saucer to the uterine wall, and to the developing fetus via the umbilical cord. It is through the placenta, which is rich in blood vessels, that all nutrients pass from the mother to the fetus; in turn, fetal waste products pass through the placenta back to the mother.

As the placenta grows during pregnancy, it also produces correspondingly greater quantities of estrogen and progesterone, a function which makes it central to the DES story.

The progesterone made by the placenta maintains the uterus as a suitable environment for the growing fetus, and appears to suppress ovulation. Progesterone is broken down in the body to an inactive substance called pregnanediol, which is excreted in the urine. By measuring the amount of pregnanediol in the urine, it is possible to estimate the amount of progesterone being produced.

## Testes

The testes (or testicles) are to the male what the ovaries are to the female. The testicles are the major producers of testosterone, which is comparable in its effects on the male to estrogen's effects on the female. The testicles also produce sperm. (A small amount of testosterone is also produced in the adrenal glands.)

The cells responsible for producing testosterone, called the interstitial cells, are not present in the child, but *are* present in the male infant, and reappear at puberty to remain throughout life. The presence of testosterone-producing tissue in the infant attests to the need for male hormone in the proper development of the male organs before birth.

The resumption of testosterone production at puberty causes the penis, scrotal sacs, and testes to enlarge many times. It also causes the growth of hair on the body and decreased growth of hair on the head. As testosterone production continues, the voice deepens, the skin becomes thicker and more rugged, with more pigment than in the female, bones grow and thicken, muscles develop and strengthen greatly by comparison to the female musculature, and the general rate of metabolism is increased, sometimes by as much as 30 percent (which may help to explain how teenaged boys can eat so much without getting fat!).

If little or no testosterone is present during fetal development, or theoretically, if large quantities of estrogen counteract the effects of the male hormone, several abnormal conditions may result. These include nonfunctional testes, undeveloped testes and penis, or undescended testes. If a boy loses his testicles, either by accident, disease, or surgery, before puberty, he becomes a eunuch, a neutered male with none of the secondary sexual features of the mature male. The effects of castration on the immature male animal have long been used to economic advantage by farmers to produce more docile, meatier, and more tender-fleshed creatures (the gelding, the steer, and the capon).

In some European countries, especially during the Middle Ages but done through the nineteenth century, it was not an unusual practice to castrate boy sopranos solely to preserve their clear, high voices! (One wonders if the castratos themselves found the career worth the price.)

## Adrenal Glands

The adrenal glands are of interest in the DES story because the outer shell, or *cortex*, of these two glands produces a group of steroids known as the corticosteroids, which are amazingly similar in chemical structure to the sex hormones. The common chemical precursor of the corticosteroids, as well as of progesterone and testosterone, is cholesterol, a substance commonly thought of as a biological villain, but which is, in fact, necessary to our well-being.

The adrenals also produce small amounts of testosterone and progesterone, so it is not surprising to learn that the adrenals share a common embryonic tissue origin with the ovaries and the testicles.

## Pancreas

This largest of all endocrine glands produces insulin. Too little or no insulin secretion results in diabetes. Interestingly, the injection of large quantities of estrogen (and theoretically, DES) can elevate blood sugar to the point of producing a diabetic-like condition in the pancreas, yet another illustration of how interactive and interdependent the endocrine system is.

## Thyroid

If the pituitary gland is the master gland that signals the other endocrine glands when and how to work, then the thyroid gland may be compared to a dynamo or energizer.

The hormones produced in this butterfly-shaped organ regulate metabolism, the process whereby food is used by the body and converted into energy. Metabolism occurs in every cell of the body.

If the thyroid gland slows down its production of hormone in childhood, cretinism results. In extreme cases, growth is slowed down to the point where a 17-year-old may be indistinguishable in appearance from a five-year-old, and intelligence is blunted to the point of profound retardation. The cells in the body simply do not have the energy to function, to grow, and to regenerate.

If the thyroid gland produces too little hormone in adulthood, *hypo*thyroidism results. As in cretinism, bodily functions go into a kind of slow motion, as the thyroid or "dynamo" slows its production of "energizer." The adult with hypothyroidism suffers from extreme and constant fatigue, swollen eyelids, hands, and feet, poor wound healing, an inability to properly metabolize fats, a reduction in the total blood volume, the blunting of intelligence, and possibly severe anemia.

In the March 14, 1977, issue of the *Journal of the American*

*Medical Association* (*JAMA*), there was an article that made an association between pregnancy and thyroid malfunctioning. The authors suggested that postpartum depression, the "blues" many women suffer following the birth of a baby, was a symptom of a painless thyroiditis, or inflammation of the thyroid. Although the reasons for this inflammation were not given, the typical postpartum thyroiditis was described as beginning with an overproduction (hyperthyroidism) of thyroid hormone and ending, four to six months after delivery, in hypothyroidism. A small number of women, they said, became permanently hypothyroid, just as I did.

Is this postpartum thyroiditis somehow caused by the sudden drop in estrogen when pregnancy terminates? Could the abrupt cessation of very high doses of DES toward the end of my own pregnancy have sent my own thyroid into a permanent depression? While this cannot be proved, it seems a possibility.

As the endocrine glands exert their effects on the body, the pituitary—the "master gland"—keeps them all in balance through a kind of push-pull effect.

For example, if a normal healthy person receives extra thyroid hormone, either by pill or injection, the pituitary compensates for this overload by decreasing its production of thyroid-stimulating (thyrotropic) hormone. If this process continues over a period of time, the thyroid gland can permanently lose its ability to secrete hormone because of chronic lack of stimulation from the pituitary. So, in response to an overload of thyroid hormone, the pituitary will have restored hormonal balance by suppressing the thyroid gland, even to the point of its destruction.

This regulatory effect of the pituitary has been well-known since the 1930s. It is not unreasonable, then, to assume that overloads of other hormones (or hormonelike substances, such as DES) could cause the pituitary to respond by increasing or decreasing corresponding hormones.

In the 1930s and 40s, a number of scientific papers reported the results of injecting large quantities of estrogen into healthy animals. Scientists found that such injections caused, among other things, an overgrowth of the adrenal cortex by somehow stimulating the pituitary to produce too much ACTH.

## • ABOUT DES IN PARTICULAR

Could DES, the "imposter" estrogen, cause similar untoward effects?

A good deal of what was written about DES in the 10 years or so following its discovery indicates that it acted amazingly like the real, natural estrogen. So accepted did DES become as "estrogen" that even in the mid-1950s, a widely respected textbook on physiology by Arthur C. Guyton, M.D., equated DES with the natural hormones. Over the title "Chemical Formulae of the Principal Female Sex Hormones," Guyton showed five chemical molecular structures: those of the three natural estrogens, progesterone, *and* DES. That DES was synthetic was given such minor consideration that the reader is left to make his or her own way to the next page, there to find DES properly identified. Despite this blanket acceptance of DES, Dr. Guyton acknowledged two significant differences between DES and the natural estrogen: that DES is much more potent and that DES is not destroyed by gastric secretions the way natural estrogen is.

This paradox in Dr. Guyton's book—acceptance of DES as the real thing even while noting important differences—merely reflected general scientific and medical thinking during those years. But, here, we are getting ahead of our story. Let us go back to the beginning, to when DES was first discovered.

### DES Is Discovered

DES was introduced to the world in 1938 by Sir E. Charles Dodds, a professor of biochemistry at the University of London.

The development of DES was, without doubt, a climactic event in sex hormone research. For two and a half decades before the development of DES, scientists had labored to define, measure, purify, and apply to medical use the biologically active substance first extracted from the ovaries in 1912. The substance, which we now know as estrogen, was called "estrus-producing hormone" for its ability to produce sexual-menstrual cycles in spayed female animals.

An abiding interest had been established in hormone therapy during the preceding several decades as diseases caused by hormone deficiencies became recognized. Diabetes, hypothyroidism, and Addison's disease are just a few of the more prominent conditions traced to hormone deficiencies during those years.

Deficiencies in estrogen were also recognized as causing abnormal conditions, as one could plainly see, for example, following the surgical removal of the ovaries. The search for ways to replace the deficient hormones had gotten underway. And by the close of the 1920s, the first nearly pure estrogen had been prepared by Edward Doisy, an American scientist who later won the Nobel Prize for Medicine.

Over the following decade, research into sex hormones has been described as a history of the work of one man—Sir E. Charles Dodds.

Working in the Courtauld Laboratory of the University of London, Dodds and his associates produced scores of papers, including those on the impact of sex hormones on the clinical practice of gynecology and obstetrics. Dodds's discovery in 1934 of the first artificial estrogen was the first evidence that compounds chemically different from natural estrogens could have the estrus-producing effect. The chemical groundwork was thus laid for the discovery of DES four years later.

Dodds's introduction of DES in 1938 was greeted with a frenzy of enthusiasm, and within two and a half years, more than 250 papers on this new drug had been written. Dodds had succeeded in developing the first easily manufactured, easily administered, and inexpensive estrogen. By contrast, the natural hormone was difficult and expensive to extract in pure form, almost impossible to standardize for potency, and was troublesome to administer to patients. The natural hormone had to be injected to be effective since its potency was almost entirely destroyed by gastric juices when it was taken by mouth. DES, on the other hand, remained extremely potent when taken orally.

For a medical community enamored with the biological power of hormones, but still too inexperienced with them to comprehend their limitations and dangers, DES was a fascinating addition to its stock of remedies.

Paralleling the events leading to the development of DES were the careers of two Harvard doctors, the husband-and-wife, physician-and-biochemist, team of Dr. George Van Siclen Smith and Dr. Olive Watkins Smith. The Smiths' professional interest had always been the ovary and its functions and interactions with the pituitary gland. Both doctors had impeccable academic credentials: he was a graduate of Harvard Medical School and she had a Ph.D. from Radcliffe. The Smiths were highly intelligent and hard-working, and their work was taken seriously.

The Smiths started administering naturally derived estrogen to pregnant women as early as 1938, prophetically the same year that DES was developed. Four years earlier they had reported their observation that the amounts of estrogen in the blood and urine of pregnant women dropped at least four or more weeks before the occurrence of complications late in pregnancy, such as toxemia, premature delivery, and death of the fetus.

In 1937, using a newly developed technique for measuring pregnanediol (the metabolic by-product of progesterone) in urine, they published their findings that this hormone, too, decreased before complications of late pregnancy set in. In 1939, another group of doctors reported similar decreases in estrogen and progesterone prior to early pregnancy miscarriage. Thus, the stage was set for hormone treatment in pregnancy.

The rationale for using DES, as opposed to the natural hormones, began with yet another set of the Smiths' observations. Again, by measuring hormones and hormone by-products in the blood and urine of pregnant women, they had observed that a rise in estrogen always seemed to precede a rise in progesterone, the hormone responsible for preparing and maintaining a woman's body for pregnancy. They concluded that estrogen, working through the pituitary, caused an increased secretion of progesterone from the placenta. We know now that the presence of estrogen *is* essential to the production of progesterone.

Now keep in mind the "push-pull" effect characteristic of the whole endocrine system. The Smiths also wrote that when the level of progesterone rose roughly in proportion to the amount of estrogen in the body, the pituitary balanced the amount of hormones by ceasing to stimulate any further production of progesterone.

Then the Smiths discovered something very interesting. They observed a marked difference in the biological effects of natural estrogen and DES. But instead of being suspicious, they were triumphant.

They had found in DES an estrus-producing substance that, unlike the natural estrogen, would apparently go right on stimulating the pituitary to spur progesterone production in the placenta, *no matter how much progesterone was already present!* In effect, they found that DES could allegedly upset and bypass the balancing effect of the pituitary.

So was born the reason for using DES to treat threatened pregnancies. DES was to be used, not for its direct estrogenic effects, but because it appeared to stimulate the body's own production of progesterone, which is necessary to sustain pregnancy.

The Smiths were to write many years later that "our purpose in recommending the prophylactic [preventive] administration of diethylstilbestrol" was to stimulate the placenta to produce more of its own progesterone and "thus perhaps to forestall [pregnancy] complications."

Pooling the observations of 117 obstetricians from 16 different states throughout the country who gave DES to a total of 632 pregnant women, Dr. Olive Smith published her landmark report, which started the wholesale use of DES. The report, which appeared in the November 1948 issue of the influential *American Journal of Obstetrics and Gynecology,* claimed that DES given in increasing dosages starting at the seventh week of pregnancy and continuing until the thirty-fifth week could increase the chance for a successful pregnancy in: (1) women who had suffered one or more previous miscarriages, (2) women who had high blood pressure, (3) women who had diabetes, and (4) that *if given prophylactically (i.e., as a preventive measure)* could protect against complications occurring late in pregnancy such as toxemia and eclampsia.

In other words, the Smiths were recommending that high doses of a drug be given *before* there was any evidence of trouble, or any sign that treatment was needed.

During the next five years, obstetricians from all over the country enthusiastically responded by prescribing millions of milligrams of DES to hundreds of thousands of pregnant women. It is estimated that most of the two to three million pregnant women who received DES were treated in the late 1940s and early 1950s.

Apparently, none of the prescribing physicians questioned the absence of a "control" group of women in the Smith study. A control group is composed of individuals similar in every relevant way to the test group, except that the controls are not exposed to the substance or condition being tested; a control group is considered essential by today's scientific standards.

Also, the 117 obstetricians participating in the Smith study had no standardized criteria to follow in caring for their 632 patients, except for a very precise dosage schedule of DES. In spite of these major flaws, the study had a profound impact.

With an estimated one out of every five pregnancies ending in miscarriage, it is easy to understand how doctors felt under pressure to "do something" when a worried patient reported staining in early pregnancy. It was beguilingly easy for doctors to have concrete treatment to offer worried patients. It was just as easy for anxious patients to accept the substantive comfort of a daily pill. DES was a painless, inexpensive, easy promise of success—in short, a "perfect" treatment.

Those charmed by the seemingly wondrous properties of DES paid scant attention to the report published in a French medical journal in 1938 that DES caused mammary tumors in male mice, a phenomenon confirmed two years later by two American scientists. Nor did they appear to be concerned with the numerous papers demonstrating the toxic effects of DES, especially on the livers of experimental animals, nor to the report that showed that DES fed to experimental mice *prevented* implantation of a fertilized ovum and resulted in abnormal degeneration of the corpus luteum, nor to the study by a Northwestern University Medical School group, which showed intersexual changes (male to female and female to male) in the DES-exposed offspring of rats fed the drug in pregnancy.

The Smiths themselves disavowed the reports of toxicity by stating that only nine of the 632 women in their study developed any side effects, and these, they said, were relatively minor. Furthermore, they expressed doubt that these side effects were attributable to DES and stated that "probably only the rare case [woman] will not be able to tolerate the full dosage schedule [of DES] throughout [pregnancy]."

Undoubtedly, much of the confidence displayed in the Smiths' work was engendered by their lofty positions in the medical community, Harvard being considered "tops" by many people and the Smiths being "tops" at Harvard. Dr. George Smith was chairman of the Department of Gynecology at Harvard Medical School for nearly two and a half decades, from 1942 to 1967. And, both Olive and George were nationally recognized and respected for their work in demonstrating and quantitating hormones during pregnancy.

But some of the confidence was motivated by a curious brand of team spirit.

"As a former Bostonian," averred Dr. Frederick Irving of Clearwater, Florida, "I would be entirely lacking in civic loyalty if I had not used stilbestrol in my private practice." That physicians practice the teachings of their local medical gurus is not so surprising.

But this affinity toward DES because of regional association of the physician has, in fact, a firmer base than the statement of a single physician. The geographical usage patterns of DES were analyzed and published in August 1972 by the Boston Collaborative Drug Surveillance Program of Boston University Medical Center. The report states that "it is interesting to note that there was regional variation [in the use of DES]," and that there were significantly more prescriptions for the drug written in the East and Midwest than there were in the South and West, with by far the most prescriptions being written at the Boston Lying-In Hospital, the Smiths' hospital.

In all fairness, many physicians (and I count my own obstetrician among them) were motivated by a genuine desire to help their patients have a successful pregnancy. And the Smiths' argument for using DES was persuasive. After all, what could be simpler? If hormone levels that should be high are found to be low and it has been seen that low levels antecede miscarriage, what could be more logical than giving a drug that makes those levels rise again? It was seductively simple.

For all the bland acceptance of DES use in pregnancy, most startling of all was the absence of concern that the Smiths had done most of their DES experiments on humans! Specifically, on women. But in fact, human experimentation without benefit of informed consent seemed to be the order of the day. Any doctor with an idea and a sufficient number of patients could experiment. And like marchers in search of a parade, doctors went in search of new medical uses for DES.

A casual perusal of the medical literature of the early 1940s uncovered a chilling number of trial-and-error medical experiments using DES on women.

In one such experiment, a doctor used large doses of DES dissolved in milk in an effort to relieve the vaginitis of congenital gonorrhea in baby girls.

Another doctor used up to 720 milligrams (more than 700 times the amount of estrogen used in modern-day birth control pills) in a vain attempt to induce labor in women during their ninth month of pregnancy.

Yet a third obstetrician working in the Baltimore City Hospital in 1940 sought to discover "what effects, if any, diethylstilbestrol would exhibit on the puerperal uterus." (The puerperium is the period immediately following the termination of pregnancy, either by normal delivery or by abortion.) This doctor and his colleagues administered varying and experimental doses of DES to 200 consecutive patients who were uninformed, unaware, and unlucky. During the second week following delivery and daily DES administration, the doctors biopsied the uteruses of at least 30 of the women before giving up due to unfruitful findings, and the possibility of perforating the uterine wall. There was no pretense of concern that this procedure might be of benefit to their patients, and only incidental concern that it might be harmful.

Even in the light of the prevailing medical practices and attitudes of the 1930s and 40s, it is chilling nonetheless to read the introduction to *Women and the Crisis in Sex Hormones,* by Barbara Seaman and Gideon Seaman, M.D. The Seamans quoted Dr. Olive Smith as saying, "We have always done our work with human material. We've used animals, of course, but we thought human material was the most interesting." Dr. Smith made this remarkable statement in 1976!

The flood of DES washing through American womanhood

might have remained unchecked for many years more but for two investigations into the effectiveness of DES in maintaining pregnancy.

The results of the first were presented in the fall of 1952. Dr. James Henry Ferguson of Tulane University questioned the absence of controls in Dr. Olive Smith's study. So, to satisfy himself that DES was effective for the stated purpose, he administered DES to nearly 200 pregnant women, while a similar group of about the same number of women received placebos. Ferguson found that not only was DES not effective, but that the DES group actually had a slightly higher incidence of premature births and miscarriages!

Close on the heels of the Ferguson study came the Dieckmann study. Dr. William J. Dieckmann, chief of the University of Chicago's Lying-In Hospital, was also troubled by the Smith omission of control patients, so he and his colleagues went one step further than Dr. Ferguson. The Chicago study was the first controlled, *double-blind* study of the effectiveness of DES in preventing miscarriage and other pregnancy complications.

A double-blind study is one in which neither the doctor nor the patient knows who is receiving the active drug and who the placebo. A third party, often the pharmacist, dispenses the drugs and keeps a coded record. The purpose of such a study is to ensure unbiased and equal treatment of all the patients—both those who receive the test treatment and those who don't (the controls). The Seamans make the point (as did Dieckmann and his colleagues) that the 632 women in the Smith study may well have received far more attentive care from their collective 117 doctors *just because they were part of the study,* and that this special care alone may have been the reason for fewer problems.

The second basic reason for a controlled, double-blind study is to eliminate the possibility that factors *other* than the test drug might be responsible for observed changes. To eliminate psychological factors, the control group must receive a placebo, or "sugar pill," as alike in appearance as possible to the test drug, so that even the individuals in the study don't know if they are getting "the real thing."

By these criteria, the Dieckmann study was the only valid study to date of DES's effectiveness in preventing miscarriage and the complications of late pregnancy.

To ensure that their study would be *statistically significant* (that is, that there would be a sufficient number of patients so that the results couldn't be ascribed to chance or coincidence), Dr. Dieckmann and his colleagues decided to study 2,000 consecutively registered women in their prenatal clinic at the Chicago Lying-In Hospital. The study was conducted in 1952 and 1953.

Each patient was told that the tablets might help prevent pregnancy complications, and that they would not hurt either the woman or her baby. It is interesting to note that although the Dieckmann group had serious questions about the value of DES, even *they* did not question its safety.

What they did question was the underlying theory of the Smiths' recommended use of DES, namely, that DES could stimulate the placenta to secrete progesterone and estrogen, and what Dieckmann considered "the most serious criticism of the study," the Smiths' omission of a control group of women.

As to the Smiths' theory that pregnancy complications could be precipitated by a deficiency of placental hormones, which could be corrected by stimulating the placenta with daily doses of DES, Dieckmann wrote that "this interesting concept of the Smiths has lacked confirmation by other investigators."

Dieckmann also stressed the importance of an adequate control group, writing "a properly conducted clinical trial demands (1) that patients and staff should have no knowledge of the medication on trial; (2) that a similar group of patients should receive placebo medication which is not discernible from the medication on trial; and (3) that the two groups of patients must be treated simultaneously and as nearly alike as possible."

Of course, the Smiths' studies of DES had not met even a single one of these criteria.

The results of the Dieckmann study, an epochal event in the DES story, revealed that DES given according to the Smith regimen did not reduce the number of miscarriages, premature or postmature births, nor did it decrease the incidence of late-pregnancy complications such as toxemia or eclampsia. As a matter of fact, the group of women who had taken DES suffered a slightly higher number of miscarriages.

When the Dieckmann results were reported at the annual meeting of the American Gynecologic Society in the spring of 1953, both Drs. Smith and their supporters were indignant, claiming that the Chicago study was not comparable to their studies and that Dr. Dieckmann and his colleagues had misunderstood them!

During the discussion following the presentation of Dr. Dieckmann's paper, Dr. George Smith who, with his wife, was in the audience, emphatically repudiated the findings of the Chicago group.

"The negative results just reported," he argued, "and those recently published by Dr. Ferguson mean to us that not enough heterogeneous pregnancies were studied." He failed to mention that the Smiths' own claims were based on fewer than half the number of women than in the Chicago study.

Dr. Smith went on to reaffirm his confidence that DES had "saved many babies."

"We trust," he concluded, "that the many obstetricians who have been following our recommendations . . . will realize that the paper presented this morning and the report by Dr. Ferguson fail to provide definite evidence to the contrary [of the Smith claims]."

Mirroring her husband's unyielding confidence in their own assertions about DES, Dr. Olive Smith insisted that scientists, including Dr. Dieckmann, whose findings differed from their own had "misrepresented" the Smiths' work and had failed "to realize the importance of following the procedures adopted by us." No mention was made of the fact that the Smiths' procedures as well as their claims were being challenged.

There seems no doubt that the Smiths were convinced that DES could "save babies." But their refusal to attribute *any* validity to a study as carefully conceived as Dieckmann's leaves one wondering if intellectual conviction hadn't been flawed just a bit by ego.

The following year, in August 1954, in a paper published in the medical journal *Obstetrics and Gynecology*, the Smiths reaffirmed their belief that DES was beneficial. Titled "Prophylactic Hormone Therapy," their paper urged the institution of *preventive* DES therapy in high-risk women as soon as pregnancy was diagnosed.

In spite of the Smiths' insistence that DES treatment was effective, the Dieckmann study did have an impact. The message that DES didn't work began to sink in and the number of prescriptions written for pregnant women began to decline, and by the last half of the 1960s, it is estimated that less than one percent of pregnancies seen at the Boston Lying-In Hospital were being treated with DES.

But, although the prescription of DES for pregnant women declined greatly during the 1960s, it did not stop altogether until 1971, a full 18 years after the Dieckmann report.

After the unquestioned administration of DES to millions of women, using the drug had become something of an obstetrical crutch, and crutches—once you get used to them—are hard to throw away.

## DES—The Die-Hard

In spite of the fact that the Food and Drug Administration has outlawed the use of DES during pregnancy, DES is still being prescribed for women in vast quantities.

In 1972 Doris Haire wrote in *The Cultural Warping of Childbirth* that "more than 40 million women have been given DES as a lactation suppressant." Now, nearly 10 years later, DES continues to be prescribed to dry up milk in new mothers who do not wish to nurse.

It is also being prescribed for thousands of young women in the form of the morning-after birth control pill. The trouble with this pill is that many of the women given this treatment (the morning-after pill is really a series of pills given over a five-day period) are probably not even pregnant. And if they are, even one missed pill can render the treatment ineffective, and should abortion be rejected, more DES babies can be born.

DES is also given to relieve the symptoms of menopause (although it and other estrogens have been linked to an increased incidence of cervical cancer and endometrial cancer—cancer of the uterine lining), as replacement therapy for women who have had their ovaries surgically removed, and as a treatment for women with advanced cases of breast cancer and for men with prostate cancer (even though DES has been associated with the development of breast cancer in these men).

Like the cancer it can cause, DES is proving itself tough to eliminate.

# 3·The Cancer Connection

*"Says Nature to Physic what pity that we,*
*Who ought to be friends, should so seldom agree."*

*Nature and Physic, Professional*
*Anecdotes, 1835*

Mary was a typical DES patient—young, active, and getting on with her life. She was 21 years old, a recent honors graduate of college, and a member of her school's swim team. She was attractive, vivacious, and the "picture of health" when her doctor diagnosed a persistent vaginal discharge as being caused by DES-related adenocarcinoma.

"It was the most horrible day of my life," she recalled. Mary, like other young DES daughters with adenocarcinoma, underwent a radical hysterectomy, including removal of her fallopian tubes and some lymph nodes, and removal of her cancerous vagina. Surgeons also cut out part of her colon, which they used to reconstruct a vagina for her.

Mary's recovery was considered rapid. Still, she suffered. Fear of cancer, pain associated with her vaginal and abdominal surgery, and grief at the knowledge that she would never bear children were all in attendance. She was plagued with intestinal gas, a common problem in patients who have undergone intestinal surgery, and a heavy mucus discharge from her neo-vagina. She had to learn self-catheterization because of surgically induced inadequate bladder contractions, a condition she was told was temporary, but which lasted for more than half a year. And she had to accustom herself to inserting a rigid, plastic, tamponlike instrument into her neo-vagina once each day to prevent scar tissue from forming and constricting it.

Although fewer than two out of every 1,000 DES daughters develop DES-caused vaginal adenocarcinoma, more than 90 percent of all DES daughters do have benign abnormalities that require continuing medical surveillance—in itself, a never-ending reminder that the physical devastation and mental anguish that Mary suffered can strike *any* DES daughter.

As other diseases that once ravaged mankind have been brought under control and conquered, cancer has emerged as a leading cause of suffering, and death. In a very real sense, cancer has become our "black plague." Unfortunately, it took nothing short of this "plague" to stop the useless prescription of DES for pregnant women.

## The First DES Cancers in Humans Are Identified

Eighteen years after the Dieckmann study showed that DES was ineffective in preventing miscarriage, and 33 years after a French scientist showed that DES could induce the formation of cancer in mice, DES was found to cause cancer in humans.

Two doctors at the famed Massachusetts General Hospital in Boston (like the Smiths' Boston Lying-In, Massachusetts General is also associated with Harvard) had seen seven patients between 1966 and 1969 with a rare form of vaginal cancer known as clear-cell adenocarcinoma (*adeno* meaning "glandular"). This cancer had previously been reported only sporadically, and then in older women. So the occurrence of seven cases in three years was a startling event.

Even more puzzling, all seven Boston patients were young—between the ages of 14 and 24 years. Up to that time, only three cases of this vaginal cancer had ever been reported in young women.

The clustering of so many cases of such a rare disease "inevitably aroused suspicion," wrote Dr. Howard Ulfelder who, with fellow obstetrician Arthur Herbst, treated the seven young women. The doctors began searching for a common denominator, in the process ruling out such factors as vaginal douches, medications taken by the patients, and sex habits. It finally remained for the mother of one of the patients to suggest the DES she had taken during pregnancy as the possible culprit. She was chillingly correct.

The article reporting the DES-pregnancy–vaginal cancer association was little more than three pages long, but it eventually shattered the peace of mind of millions of women.

Although the actual number of women who received DES in the United States between 1940 and 1971 is not known, it is variously estimated at between 500,000 and three million. Dr. Herbst and his colleagues have conjectured that 10 percent of all pregnant women received DES between 1951 and 1960, with that figure dropping to less than one percent during the following decade.

By the time Drs. Herbst and Ulfelder and Dr. David Poskanzer (a medical epidemiologist) wrote of those first known cases of vaginal cancer from DES in April 1971, one thing was sure—more cases were bound to surface. And surface they did. Within months, other doctors wrote of cases of the disease they had treated, and almost all of the young cancer victims were DES daughters.

A brand new medical phenomenon had been uncovered: namely, a drug that could cross the placenta to reach the fetus and then cause serious disease two to three decades after exposure.

Even the thalidomide tragedy of the mid-sixties was different. The malformations caused by thalidomide were gross and immediate. The harm done by DES, on the other hand, didn't become manifest for decades.

"This disease complex is one of the few entirely new and previously unsuspected discoveries of the recent past," wrote Howard Ulfelder.

Suspicion had given way to confirmation of what caused the disease, and something had to be done.

## The DES Registry

What to do came in the form of a registry, a formal effort at gathering in one place information on all known cases of vaginal cancer in women born after 1940 (the year the Food and Drug Administration approved DES for human use). Keeping in mind the large number of women who were given DES and the possibility that many more cases of cancer would inevitably occur, it became critical to establish basic facts about this disease, a disease about which doctors knew almost nothing.

Before the close of 1971, Dr. Herbst and Dr. Robert Scully, a pathologist at the Massachusetts General Hospital, had established a central registry for all cases of clear-cell adenocarcinoma of the vagina and cervix. Dr. Herbst took the responsibility of reviewing all the clinical information about every case reported and Dr. Scully examined all tissue samples.

The new registry was advertised in the major gynecological-obstetrical and cancer journals, and letters were sent to doctors in major medical centers across the country to advertise the existence of the registry. Within two years, the Registry of Clear-Cell Adenocarcinoma of the Genital Tract had received data on 170 cases.

With the support of the National Cancer Institute and the American Cancer Society, by early 1980 the registry (which has since been renamed the Registry for Research on Hormonal Transplacental Carcinogenesis) had collected information on more than 420 cases of adenocarcinoma of the genital tract. It is the collective information in the registry that has illuminated the DES-cancer connection. We have learned from registry data the relative risk of a DES daughter developing adenocarcinoma (lower than originally feared), the course of the disease, including survival rates, the most effective treatments, and the peak ages of occurrence.

Cases have been reported from all parts of the United States, as well as from Australia, France, Israel, and Mexico.

However, DES was prescribed for pregnant women in other countries as well, including Spain (where an estimated 65 percent of all the DES prescriptions in Europe were written), Belgium, West Germany, Italy, the Netherlands, England, the Philippines, and many, if not all, the South American countries. There have been no cases of vaginal adenocarcinoma reported from the two European countries in which DES was *not* prescribed during pregnancy—namely, Denmark and Finland.

All reports to the registry are given voluntarily. Although good compliance in reporting new cases is claimed for American physicians, there is still no way to judge how truly the registry reflects the incidence of the disease.

The registry is located in the Chicago Lying-In Hospital— coincidentally of Dieckmann study fame—under the direction of Arthur Herbst, who moved to Chicago from Boston shortly after the registry was established. Dr. Herbst is also chairman of the Department of Obstetrics and Gynecology at the University of Chicago Medical School.

When the name of the registry was changed, the kinds of cancers it keeps track of were expanded. The registry now accepts reports of all cases of vaginal and cervical adenocarcinoma, whether or not there is a known history of DES exposure, and all cases of invasive genital cancers if the patient was exposed to *any* kind of hormone that her mother may have taken during pregnancy.

This last condition has been included, writes Dr. Herbst, because there is a possibility that steroid hormones affect the developing fetal genitals in a way similar to DES and related nonsteroid hormones.

## • WHAT HAS BEEN LEARNED FROM THE REGISTRY ABOUT ADENOCARCINOMA

Adenocarcinoma is so called because of the glandlike cells it contains. Vaginal and cervical adenocarcinomas rarely occur in nature, and when they do, they usually afflict older, post-menopausal women. As was mentioned before, only three cases of this disease were ever reported to have occurred in younger women before the use of DES.

The kind of adenocarcinoma of the genitals caused by DES is a disease of very young women. The oldest woman known to have developed it was 29; the youngest only seven.

In his most recent review of the cancer cases recorded in the registry, Dr. Herbst reports that the number of cancer cases in DES daughters rises sharply after the age of 14, remains at an irregular plateau between the ages of 17 and 21 years, then appears to fall thereafter. He also reports that younger cancer victims (under the age of 15) have a poorer chance for surviving the disease than those daughters who are in their late teens or early twenties when they develop it.

## Maternal History and Adenocarcinoma

The risk of developing cancer has been found to be inversely associated with the time during pregnancy that the mother began taking DES. In other words, the earlier in pregnancy the mother began taking DES, the greater the risk of subsequent cancer in her daughter. On the average, mothers of cancer victims began taking DES at about nine weeks, whereas mothers of girls who did not develop cancer began their DES therapy at about 13 weeks of pregnancy.

How much DES the mother took seems to matter less than when she took it. Mothers taking as much as 300 milligrams daily produced daughters who have not developed cancer, and daughters whose mothers took as little as 25 milligrams per day have developed the disease. Perhaps the most celebrated example of a small maternal dose of DES causing cancer in the daughter is the case of Joyce Bichler, the first DES daughter to win a lawsuit against the drug companies. Joyce's mother took only 25 milligrams of DES a day, and only for 12 days of her pregnancy. This total of 300 milligrams for Mrs. Bichler's entire pregnancy seems minuscule compared to the 10,000- and even 20,000-milligram total doses that many other women took.

## Survival

Once a DES daughter develops cancer, what are her chances for recovering?

Again, judging from registry information, her chances for being cured are much better than even. If the disease is caught at an early stage and the cancer primarily affects the cervix, chances are better than nine out of ten that she will be cured. If the tumor is on the vaginal wall, her chance for cure drops only slightly, to 87 percent.

But the outlook is not so good for women whose cancers have already spread to neighboring organs, such as the bladder or rectum, when their disease is first discovered. The chances for survival for these women drop to a dismal three out of ten—a mere 30 percent.

*What happens when the cancer recurs?* In about one out of every five of the registry's cancer patients, the disease recurs after the initial treatment. Most of these recurrences are found within three years of the first diagnosis, but in some women, the cancer has come back after as long as seven disease-free years. Once this cancer recurs, the chances for survival drop to four out of ten. One hopes that the chances of survival for these women will improve as methods of both diagnosis and treatment become more sophisticated.

*Oral contraceptives and the registry's patients.* In a registry report published in the *American Journal of Obstetrics and Gynecology* in December 1979, Dr. Herbst, Dr. Scully, and their colleagues compared survival between registry patients who used oral contraceptives and those who did not. They found no difference.

However, the more interesting question remains unanswered; namely, do DES daughters who use oral contraceptives have a greater risk of developing cancer than those who don't take the "Pill"?

## Pregnancy and Survival

The same Herbst report also reported no difference in the survival rates between pregnant and nonpregnant registry patients. But, as is pointed out, the number of women who developed DES-related cancer while pregnant is small—only 18.

## The Incidence of DES-Caused Cancer

Based on a report from the Mayo Clinic in 1973, DES-caused cancer was originally thought to occur in about one out of every 250 DES daughters. As the registry accumulated more information, estimates of the actual incidence became more optimistic. Now it is generally accepted that DES-caused genital cancer strikes, at most, one out of every 700 DES daughters, or 1.4 per 1,000 to 1.4 per 10,000 DES daughters. That means that no *more* than one out of every 700 DES daughters nor *fewer* than one out of every 7,000 will develop cancer. Doctors aren't sure of the precise risk, so they give this range of figures. Still, there is no doubt that this is a comforting piece of information.

## • THE ENIGMA OF THE ADENOCARCINOMA VICTIMS WHOSE MOTHERS DIDN'T TAKE DES

While some of the registry's information is comforting, and some is unsettling, yet other information it has generated is altogether mystifying.

Such is the case of the 25 percent of genital adenocarcinoma victims whose mothers apparently never took DES!

According to the December 1979 registry report, about two-thirds of young women who have contracted the DES cancer were, indeed, exposed to DES or to a related, nonsteroid hormone before they were born. Another one-tenth of victims were exposed prenatally to steroid hormones—estrogen and progesterone. But for the remaining one-quarter of young women with the disease, no *in utero* exposure to any kind of administered hormones can be demonstrated.

Dr. Herbst and others have acknowledged that this is very strange, strange because prior to the prescription of DES, only three cases of this cancer in young women were even known to occur. But since the advent of DES, and just in the last two decades, there are about 100 cases.

Is it coincidence? Or perhaps a fluke of nature? Could something other than hormones have caused this cancer? Was it possible that some of the mothers, at least, took DES during pregnancy unknowingly?

Any one or all of these theories are possible. In the first paper revealing the cancer connection by Herbst, Ulfelder, and Poskanzer, one of the eight patients they wrote about had no known exposure to hormones. And, the doctors pointed out then that factors other than prenatal hormone exposure could be causing the "DES cancer."

Eight years after that paper was published, Dr. Herbst stated, "These other factors were unknown then (in 1971) as they are now." Not a very satisfying answer, but he did admit that no one could be sure that all the cases in the registry apparently negative for DES exposure were truly negative.

"I believe it is likely," he wrote, "that some of these negative cases were exposed." In other words, some of the mothers of registry patients either did not remember or were unaware that they had been given DES. More than one DES mother has recalled her obstetrician describing as "pregnancy vitamins" what she subsequently found out was DES. It is probable that not all mothers who were subject to similar fabrications were astute enough to subsequently learn the truth.

To confuse matters even further, the line between truth and fiction was deliberately blurred by the pharmaceutical companies. At least one drug company placed an advertisement in several obstetrical journals to convince the *physician* that DES was a kind of pregnancy vitamin! The advertisement shows a gorgeously plump baby next to the words, "Now, stilbestrol with vitamins."

If her doctor was convinced DES was a kind of pregnancy "super-vitamin," how, then, was the medically unsophisticated and trusting mother-to-be to know she was taking something other than vitamins?

Another theory to help account for the mystery of the 25 percent is that some obstetricians may have deliberately falsified medical records of their DES patients to avoid legal recriminations.

Janelle Colton,* a vivacious and articulate national officer of DES Action, a national consumer organization, is the mother of two DES daughters. She has told me that her own obstetrical records contain absolutely no mention of her ever taking DES. "I would have thought I was going crazy," she said, "if my own husband—who is a pharmacist—hadn't filled the prescriptions himself, and *he* kept records!"

Both of Janelle's teenage daughters have vaginal adenosis, the typical benign abnormality caused by *in utero* exposure to DES.

Either it was deliberately omitted from Janelle's records that she took DES or it was omitted because of sloppy record keeping. Either possibility is inexcusable.

A third possibility explaining the DES-cancer victims who apparently were not DES-exposed, is the DES given to millions of food animals. During the 1940s, when the craze to find practical applications for DES was at its fevered height, someone decided to apply the hormone to agriculture. For years before that, farmers had surgically emasculated livestock to make them juicier, meatier, and faster growing, and hence more marketable as food. (*See* chapter 2, page 18.)

Following the discovery of DES, farmers found it was faster and cheaper to feminize their animals with DES. To caponize

---

*The name of this woman is fictitious to protect her privacy.

male chickens, farmers often implanted DES via a small pellet in the neck of the bird. In 1959, the Food and Drug Administration banned such implants because measurable amounts of DES were being found in the edible flesh of these birds. American farmers, however, continued for two more decades to use DES in the form of both pellets and food additives for beef cattle and sheep. The practice was not finally stopped until the FDA issued its most recent ban, effective November 1, 1979.

So, all of us—including pregnant women—who ate chicken up to 1959, and beef and lamb probably into the early 1980s (since DES is retained in the animal's body for up to six months after a DES pellet is implanted) were also receiving small doses of DES. Women who happened to eat the livers of these animals probably ingested a lot more DES, since DES is concentrated and eventually metabolized in this organ.

Was it possible for the small residues of DES in edible animal flesh to have a physiological effect on the people who ate it? Certainly, scientists working for the FDA must have thought so; otherwise why ban it? And, if DES residues could affect nonpregnant adults, is it not possible that even these small amounts could affect such an exquisitely sensitive target as the developing human fetus?

A fourth theory has been advanced to explain the relatively large number of DES-type cancer victims who have no apparent hormone exposure. Perhaps there has always been more of this cancer prevalent in young women than has been believed, and only now—with the advent of the DES registry and heightened medical awareness—have these cases come to light. Either that, or for some mysterious reason, there really *has* been an increase in the numbers of these cancers during the last two decades as compared to all of recorded medical history before that. I can use no other word than *mysterious* to describe this last possibility, since DES-knowledgeable physicians themselves are not sure how to explain it.

To make this matter even more puzzling, Dr. Ulfelder revealed that the DES-type cancer victims with no apparent hormone exposure "were heavily weighted" with *cervical* adenocarcinoma. This is in conspicuous contrast to the cancer victims with proven DES exposure who have a preponderance of *vaginal* cancers.

For now, what this all means is anybody's guess.

## • HOW DID DES CAUSE CANCER AND OTHER ABNORMALITIES?

Another matter over which there has been much speculation is *how* DES causes damage to the fetus.

Most knowledgeable researchers think that the drug works as a teratogen—an agent that produces abnormalities—and that the abnormal tissue is then predisposed later in life to developing cancer.

Dr. H.G. Hillemanns and his co-workers in West Germany published a persuasive argument for DES as a teratogen. "The final development of carcinomas," they wrote in the November 1979 issue of *Obstetrical and Gynecological Survey*, "may be due to the action of some cofactor [an independent agent that might act in concert with the main agent to produce an effect neither could cause alone] which operate on previously [DES] exposed cells . . . causing a . . . malignant . . . mutation."

This theory seems to be borne out in the case of the identical twin girls, one of whom developed vaginal adenocarcinoma and one of whom did not. Dr. Eugene Sandberg of Stanford University cared for the girls and raised the interesting thought that a virus may have triggered the cancer. Since both girls were genetically identical (with the same inborn resistances and susceptibilities) and both girls were equally and identically exposed to DES, there had to be another factor responsible for triggering cancer in just one of the twins. Dr. Sandberg finally found that the sister with cancer had a significantly higher level of antibodies to the Epstein-Barr virus, the virus that causes infectious mononucleosis. The high level of antibodies in the cancer-stricken twin indicates that she had been infected with the virus at one point, and that her body responded to this exposure by producing anti-bodies. The Epstein-Barr virus also is known to have cancer-causing capabilities in humans, according to Dr. Sandberg, and he acknowledged the possibility that this virus could have initiated cancer in the already DES-sensitized tissue. If this theory is correct, the antibodies the girl's body produced controlled the immediate disease caused by the virus, but did not protect against the virus's cancer-causing potential.

Other investigators believe that DES is a direct carcino-gen—a cancer-causing agent—with a 10- to 20-year lag time between exposure and development of the disease. It can take 20 to 30 years, for example, for an individual exposed to asbestos to develop asbestos-related lung cancer.

The work of Dr. John A. McLachlan, a toxicologist with the National Institute of Environmental Health Services seems to bear this out. He reported that as DES is chemically broken down in the body, it can react actively with other substances present to become directly carcinogenic.

Although the debate may continue about DES being a direct carcinogen versus DES as a predisposing agent, what seems certain is that DES somehow interferes with the normal development of the reproductive tract in the developing fetus. The resultant degree of deformity seems to be most depen-dent on *when* during her pregnancy a mother took DES, rather than on how long she took it or how much she took, although some studies do indicate a dose-related degree of deformity.

This kind of interference with fetal development depending on timing of drug exposure was graphically illustrated with thalidomide. The editors of *Consumer Reports* wrote in *The Medicine Show* that "If a pregnant woman took thalidomide between days 34 and 38 (of her pregnancy), the result was deformity of the fetal ears, paralysis of the facial nerve and duplication of thumbs. If she took thalidomide between days

39 and 44, the result was shortening of the arms . . . between days 42 and 45 . . . shortening of the legs."

With DES exposure, abnormalities (including cancer) are not found in girls whose mothers first took DES after the twentieth week of pregnancy, when the formation of the vagina and cervix are complete.

According to the registry report published in December 1979, the chance for a DES daughter to develop vaginal or cervical cancer is greater to a statistically significant degree if her mother started taking DES *before* the tenth week of pregnancy. Comparing the DES starting times of mothers of cancer patients from the registry with the starting times of mothers of DES daughters in the National Cancer Institute's DES surveillance project (DESAD; *see* chapter 7, page 124), Dr. Herbst found that, on the average, the registry patients had been exposed starting at an age of 9.2 fetal weeks, as compared to 12.8 fetal weeks of those daughters who did not get cancer.

Bear in mind, though, that these figures are just averages and, as is true for any average, there are many exceptions. Young women with a fetal exposure weeks later than the average 9.2 have developed adenocarcinoma, and conversely, thousands of young women whose mothers began taking the drug as early as the fifth week of pregnancy have *not* developed cancer.

## • HOW THE HUMAN VAGINA DEVELOPS

To better understand *why* timing of DES exposure is important, it helps to know how the human vagina is formed.

Generally, it is believed that the vagina begins to develop during the second month of pregnancy and is completed by about the fifth month, or twentieth week. Early in fetal development, tissue called columnar epithelium is present. This tissue derives from a bit of the embryo called the müllerian duct. Columnar epithelium is found in normal adult women around and just inside the cervical opening, and also lining the uterine walls. Many small, mucus-producing glands can be found in columnar epithelium. (Recall, here, that the *adeno* of adenocarcinoma means "glandular.")

As vaginal development proceeds, a new kind of tissue in the form of a solid core or vaginal "plate" begins to grow upward toward the early müllerian, columnar epithelium, eventually undermines it, and finally forms the normal vaginal canal. This new tissue is called squamous (rhymes with *famous*) epithelium and is found as the normal lining of the mature vagina.

A Norwegian scientist, John-Gunnar Forsberg, who has recreated in mice a similar phenomenon to human adenosis, has suggested that DES acts by inhibiting the growth of the vaginal plate, thereby promoting the persistence of the more primitive glandular epithelium in the vagina.

The presence of this glandular epithelium in the vagina and on the cervix is what is commonly called *adenosis*, the benign abnormality found in almost all DES daughters.

Adenosis is, in effect, misplaced tissue. A Department of Health, Education, and Welfare brochure compares adenosis to the lining inside our mouths. Adenosis in the vagina is as if the lining inside our mouths grew out onto our lips and cheeks.

## The Transformation Zone—Breeding Ground for Cancer?

If this tissue called adenosis is not abnormal, but merely abnormally placed, then why the worry?

Well, besides the obvious reason that adenosis has been found in virtually every DES daughter with vaginal or cervical cancer, it is a kind of tissue that undergoes rapid change. At puberty and later in DES daughters, when adenosis is exposed to the more acidic vaginal environment of the maturing woman, it undergoes conversion by the process called *metaplasia* to squamous epithelium, the tissue normally found lining the vagina. Metaplasia is a rapid, but essentially normal process whereby tissue changes from one form to another.

The glandular epithelium outside of the cervix (the adenosis) is called the *transformation zone*. All women normally have a small transformation zone of varying sizes around the cervical opening. This transformation zone tissue has a greater susceptibility to convert to cancer. The reason for this, perhaps, is that because of orderly but rapid (metaplastic) changes this tissue undergoes, the opportunity for disorderly or *dysplastic* (precancerous) or *neoplastic* (cancerous) change is greater. According to an article in the November 1979 issue of *Obstetrical and Gynecological Survey*, metaplasia does, indeed, have a "well-known high sensitivity to cancer."

In DES daughters, the amount of metaplastic tissue (i.e., the transformation zone) is simply much larger than in nonexposed women, hence, the apparent increased risk for developing cancer.

*The squamo-columnar junction.* Another way of discussing the transformation zone is by referring to the squamo-columnar junction—the border at which the normal, squamous epithelium of the vagina meets the columnar epithelium normally found in and around the mouth of the cervix. The lower down in the vagina the squamo-columnar junction is, the larger the transformation zone.

*Adenosis recedes.* As the metaplastic process (the conversion during which adenosis changes to normal squamous epithelium) continues, theoretically, we should expect adenosis to disappear. And, in fact, this is what appears to happen as young women enter their mid- and late twenties.

During the past decade, as tens of thousands of DES daughters have been examined, doctors have observed that the transformation zone or area of adenosis shrinks, or "heals," as columnar epithelium is replaced by normal vaginal squamous epithelium. This observation was confirmed by Drs. Donald Antonioli and Louis Burke of Boston's Beth Israel Hospital in their paper on the natural regression of DES-associated benign abnormalities, which was published in the August 1, 1980 issue of the *American Journal of Obstetrics and Gynecology.*

As squamous epithelium replaces the adenosis, the chances of a DES daughter developing adenocarcinoma are presumed to decrease. This assumption appears to be borne out by the statistics available from the registry, which show that the number of cases of adenocarcinoma do drop significantly in DES daughters 24 years old and older.

However, there is a chance that underneath the newly formed layer of squamous epithelium, glandular tissue can persist, perhaps still with a heightened susceptibility to developing cancer. In a 1977 symposium on DES sponsored by the American College of Obstetricians and Gynecologists, Dr. Robert Scully, chief pathologist for the registry, acknowledged this could happen. "A rare carcinoma has been confined to the lamina propria," he reported, "and covered by the squamous epithelium of the vagina or cervix."

In other words, in spite of the fact that the surface layer of tissue could appear normal, a cancer might still grow beneath the surface which would require careful palpation—and not just a Pap smear—to detect.

## • OTHER CANCERS?

Although vaginal and cervical adenocarcinoma have been the central focus of the DES issue, there is a possibility that DES daughters may be at risk for other cancerous and precancerous changes of the cervix and vagina.

Such changes are often loosely grouped under the term *dysplasia*, which covers the gamut of disorderly cell changes from mild (noncancerous) to severe (precancerous). *Neoplasia* includes tissue that has already begun to turn cancerous, as well as indisputably malignant tissue. Some doctors are now using these terms interchangeably, but the definitions I have just given are scientifically correct. The distinction between severe dysplasia and neoplasia is frequently a blurry one, and the reported incidence of DES daughters with neoplasia varies greatly, from 1.2 percent to 18 percent.

These figures do *not* include adenocarcinoma (cancer of glandular origin), but, rather, refer to neoplasia of the squamous epithelium, the tissue newly formed by metaplasia. Unlike adenocarcinoma, this neoplasia is generally *noninvasive*. In other words, it remains superficial and does not spread for periods of up to 10 years following its development, whereas adenocarcinoma spreads quickly to invade neighboring tissues, even when the original tumor is still quite small.

This superficial, squamous neoplasia is generally referred to as cancer *in situ* (meaning cancer that stays "in place").

The possibility that DES daughters might be at increased risk for developing these noninvasive, superficial neoplasias has been the subject of debate among experts.

Dr. Adolph Stafl, regarded as one of the foremost colposcopy experts in the country, is a proponent of the theory that DES daughters may be developing more *in situ* carcinomas than their DES-unexposed sisters.

In a telephone interview, Dr. Stafl told me he bases his opinion on his own clinical experience at the Medical College of Wisconsin in Milwaukee, and on a collection of data from 35 cases of DES-associated neoplasias in part referred to him by other gynecologists and pathologists.

He said that what he found was a very big difference in the microscopic interpretations of tissue sample between different pathologists, all of whom were experts. Dr. Stafl admitted that there is no consensus on the relative risk of neoplasia in DES daughters. He offered three reasons for this lack of agreement.

One reason, he said, is that the patient population from which one infers conclusions is different from doctor to doctor. In other words, the incidence of neoplasia is likely to be higher in a group of patients who have sought medical attention because of symptoms than in a nonsymptomatic, random group of DES daughters.

The second reason is that different pathologists give different interpretations to the same biopsied tissue samples. Dr. Ralph Richart of Columbia University's College of Physicians and Surgeons agrees that there is no consensus among pathologists about tissue samples, but believes that these differences of opinion are more than just experts disagreeing. He writes that "there is a tendency to overdiagnose DES-related epithelial lesions both clinically and histopathologically." Overdiagnosis in this sense means that the doctor interprets an abnormal tissue sample as being *more* diseased or as being closer to a cancerous state than is really the case. He says that many doctors may interpret abnormal-looking tissue as *neo*plasia when all it is, is immature *meta*plasia. Dr. Richart believes that there is probably *not* a statistically significant increase in DES-related neoplasias, but cautions that "a great deal of additional study must take place" before firm conclusions can be drawn about whether or not DES daughters have more *in situ* carcinomas than other women.

The third reason for disagreement, according to Dr. Stafl, is that techniques of examination differ from doctor to doctor, so that one doctor may find a severe dysplasia or neoplasia that another doctor has overlooked.

In practical terms, who is right in this debate is almost academic. Because these superficial cancers are very slow growing, regular DES check-ups are likely to detect all cases of *in situ* carcinomas in time to treat them successfully.

## Will There Be Another Wave of Adenocarcinoma?

Now for the bad news. There is a possibility of a second wave of the far more virulent and deadly adenocarcinoma.

In his review of registry cases, which was published in the December 1979 issue of the *American Journal of Obstetrics and Gynecology*, Dr. Herbst acknowledged the possibility of a "second age-incidence peak" of the disease. The first, as we know, occurs between the ages of 14 and 23 years. The second may appear in later life.

The oldest DES daughters are just now in their late thirties. No one knows what will happen as they approach their forties and fifties, ages at which the incidence of all kinds of cancer increase sharply, regardless of drug exposure, in the general population.

In the DES-*un*exposed population, invasive carcinoma of the vagina comprises about 2 percent of all female genital cancers. The mean age of women who get it is 56 years. Will the normal aging process trigger a second wave of invasive vaginal cancer in the already sensitized tissue of DES daughters?

Unfortunately, this is a question only the passage of time can answer.

# 4·The Daughters of DES

*"Since my mother had already taken DES, there was nothing I could do but get my body checked out. I realized that my getting upset and hysterical wouldn't reverse anything."*

A 16-year-old DES daughter, DES Action
Voice, *Vol. 2, No. 3, Winter 1980*

The daughters of DES are legion. They number in the millions and they have many faces. They range from grade-school age to middle age; from poor to rich; from the very naive to the hip sophisticate. They have been born in every state of the union, in big cities as well as in small towns.

Yet for all their differences, they are forged into a sisterhood—unwilling, but undeniable.

They are bonded not merely by the common fear that they *could* develop the dreaded adenocarcinoma (although relatively few have so far), but also by real physical problems. These range from minor anomalies of the genital tract to major malformations, making it difficult, and sometimes impossible, for them to bear children. In fact, pregnancy and fertility problems are proving to be the real misfortune for DES daughters.

Take Hannah, for example, a DES daughter who recently celebrated her thirtieth birthday. After four years of marriage, she and her husband were elated to find out that Hannah was pregnant. Following an adolescence and young adulthood fraught with severe menstrual problems and several years of married life enduring scores of gynecological examinations and fertility tests, the fact that Hannah had finally become pregnant seemed nothing short of miraculous.

Hannah's fertility problems had begun before she was born. In soft-spoken, well-measured words, Hannah told me that her mother had taken DES for seven of the nine months she was pregnant with Hannah. The fact that Hannah's father is a physician and allowed his wife to take DES is mute testimony to the general acceptance of DES during the late 1940s and 1950s. Hannah herself believes that most doctors who prescribed DES were well-intentioned, and feels no anger toward them.

But as a result of her mother's use of DES, Hannah has many DES-related medical problems. Although she didn't learn about her DES exposure until she was 22 years old, Hannah knew something was wrong years earlier. While most American girls start menstruating at about 13 years of age, Hannah didn't get her first period until she was 17 years old. Then, her periods came erratically, and as hemorrhagic rushes of blood accompanied by violent cramping, headaches, and vomiting. These symptoms have lessened in severity slightly over the years.

She sought medical help and was told she had a "cockscomb cervix" (*see* page 59, illustration page 60), an abnormality later found to be common in DES daughters. By the time she had endured her third period, her doctor prescribed birth control pills in an effort to regulate her system. She took them for four years and although her menstrual cycle became more regular, her violent menstrual symptoms persisted. She recalls that during this time her greatest frustration was "just getting doctors to take me seriously." She was told that it wasn't serious, and that there really wasn't anything doctors could do for her.

At age 22, when she discovered she was a DES daughter, she said she became "filled with the terror of cancer." Her mother, she said, suffered from extreme guilt.

Four years later, during a regular DES check-up, her doctor found that Hannah had a cervical carcinoma *in situ*, an early, localized, and easily curable malignancy. Carcinoma *in situ* is suspected by some doctors to occur more frequently in DES daughters (*see* chapter 3), and while it is easily treated, if left untreated, it can develop into full-blown, invasive, and life-threatening cancer. (For more on treatments, *see* last section, this chapter.)

But Hannah's DES-caused problems did not stop then. After trying, fruitlessly, to become pregnant for more than a year, she and her husband went to see a fertility specialist who put them through a routine series of tests—a medical history, a sperm count, a postcoital test (to see if her husband's sperm could survive in her vagina and uterus long enough to fertilize an ovum). When these tests revealed nothing wrong, Hannah was instructed to take her temperature rectally each morning before she got out of bed and to keep a chart of each day's reading to help determine if she was ovulating. Characteristically, there is a discernible rise in body temperature when ovulation occurs. Still, she did not conceive. After several months, the doctor did an endometrial biopsy to make sure Hannah's uterine lining was able to sustain a fertilized egg if conception should occur.

Finally, Hannah underwent a hysterosalpingogram, an x-ray procedure of the uterus and fallopian tubes, which requires an injection of large amounts of a dyelike fluid through the cervix and into the uterus and fallopian tubes. The fluid then shows up these organs as solid, white bodies on the x-ray film, thus revealing their internal contours and any irregularity or blockage.

In Hannah's case, the hysterosalpingogram revealed that her uterus was abnormally small (one-third the normal size) and abnormally shaped. In spite of this, said her doctor, Hannah could still become pregnant and deliver a child. She went home not only with severe cramping from the hysterosalpingogram, but with a growing sense of despondency.

Eight months later, when she and her husband had all but given up hope of having a child, Hannah became pregnant. The first two months of her pregnancy passed without incident. Then, during the third month, following a routine obstetrical check-up, Hannah experienced a bright red gush of vaginal bleeding. Frantic, she went back to her doctor who assured her that the pregnancy was still intact. But the bleeding episode convinced him that Hannah's obstetrical care should be taken over by a physician who specializes in high-risk pregnancies. Her obstetrician was concerned by now that Hannah—like many DES daughters—might miscarry because of an incompetent cervix. (An incompetent cervix is one that opens early in pregnancy, as soon as the weight of the womb grows great enough, so that the fetus literally drops out.) He suggested that she ask her new doctor about doing a cerclage, a simple procedure in which the cervix is stitched, which keeps it closed until the end of pregnancy.

When Hannah visited her new doctor for the first time, she asked him about doing a cerclage. He dismissed the suggestion as unwarranted. One month later, Hannah miscarried because of an incompetent cervix. Her doctor was chastened, but it was too late to save Hannah's pregnancy. At first, the pain of her loss seemed unbearable, Hannah told me. Then it was replaced by an unshakable yearning to become pregnant again, as soon as possible, but Hannah's husband doesn't want her to become pregnant again. So grief-stricken was *he* at the loss of the pregnancy that he cannot bear the thought of risking such hurt again. So for now, Hannah wrestles with two demons—her own thwarted desire to bear a child and her husband's fears of another problem pregnancy.

Andrea is another DES daughter with abnormalities of the vagina, cervix, and uterus. During the first six years of her marriage, she suffered a miscarriage, a stillbirth due to premature labor, and two ectopic (tubal) pregnancies. The tubal pregnancies necessitated removal of both her fallopian tubes, consigning her to permanent sterility by the time she was 28 years old.

## • THE BENIGN ABNORMALITIES OF THE DES DAUGHTER

Together, Hannah and Andrea have had virtually all of the common benign problems found in DES daughters. The following explanations of these abnormalities should be helpful to you in understanding your own medical findings and should help to put some fears to rest.

*Adenosis.* The most commonly found noncancerous abnormality in DES daughters is adenosis. Briefly restated (it is explained in detail in chapter 3), it consists of glandular tissue lining the *outside* of the cervix and the vagina, which in other women is found only *inside* the cervix, the uterus, and the fallopian tubes.

Estimates of the number of DES daughters with adenosis range from 30 percent to 97 percent. In the general population not exposed to DES, adenosis occurs in only about 4 percent of women. These figures are supported by a 1979 study of 281 females stillborn at the Boston Lying-In Hospital from 1946 to 1968 and whose autopsied tissues had been preserved. The study found that adenosis was present in the vaginas of 81 percent of DES-exposed fetuses, but in only 4 percent of unexposed fetuses.

Usually, adenosis causes few or no problems, although in some women it may cause heavy mucus discharges, resulting from small, mucus-producing glands in the adenosis. Other complaints have included a feeling of heat in the vagina, pain during intercourse, and abnormal vaginal bleeding. Adenosis may be tender and may bleed on contact during examination. However, the prime concern about adenosis is its unknown potential for becoming cancerous.

*Cervical ectropion.* This condition is to the cervix what adenosis is to the vagina. In other words, it is the growth of glandular tissue on the outside of the cervix. As with most cases of adenosis, the only treatment prescribed is careful and regular examinations, important because this tissue, like adenosis, may have an increased susceptibility to malignant transformation.

*Cockscomb or hooded cervix.* This is a structural anomaly which consists of a raised ridge or sometimes a complete ring of tissue around the cervix, giving it a hooded appearance (*see* illustrations). As with adenosis and cervical ectropion, the cervical cockscombs and hoods are reported to regress and in some cases to disappear as DES daughters grow older, usually by the middle to late twenties.

*Vaginal or cervical transverse ridges.* These, similar to the cockscombs or hoods found around the cervix, are abnormal ridges of tissue across the wall of the upper vagina, which is normally smooth. These ridges seem to occur more frequently in young women whose mothers took DES early in pregnancy.

*White epithelium, leukoplakia, mosaicism, punctation, and nabothian cysts.* Leukoplakia is a disturbance in the normal maturation of the squamous epithelium, and has a milky appearance; hence, the term *white epithelium.* As with other benign abnormalities, this is reported to regress and disappear as DES daughters enter their mid- and late twenties. *Mosaicism* and *punctation* are descriptive terms applied to abnormal configurations of capillaries in vaginal and cervical tissue. A mosaic pattern of blood vessels resembles a tile mosaic; punctation looks like many small, red dots which represent the endings of blood vessels. *Nabothian cysts* form in the vaginal and cervical tissue as squamous epithelium is formed through metaplasia. These cysts were originally small glands whose ducts to the surface became plugged with the newly forming squamous tissue, thus forming cysts beneath the surface. All of these conditions are noncancerous abnormalities, but still should be watched and followed by a DES-knowledgeable physician.

*Upper genital tract structural abnormalities.* Less obvious on routine examination, but probably more consequential than cervical or vaginal changes are the upper genital tract abnormalities found in DES daughters. Just as adenosis appears to be the result of arrested genital development during

## Your doctor's view of your cervix during a pelvic examination

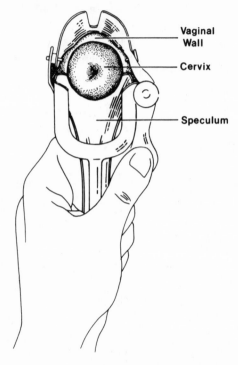

Vaginal
Wall

Cervix

Speculum

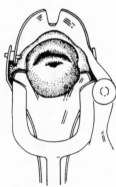

**Partially
Hooded Cervix**

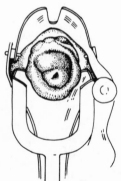

**Cockscomb with
Cleft Formation**

fetal life due to DES exposure, the uterus and fallopian tubes seem to have been similarly affected.

Careful observation has shown that DES daughters with structural abnormalities of the cervix have a 75 percent chance of also having abnormalities in the size and shape of the uterus.

Dr. Raymond Kaufman of Baylor College of Medicine in Texas and one of the medical directors of the DESAD project (the government-funded investigation of the effects of DES), was the first to report these changes. He found that 40 out of 60 DES daughters he examined in one study had abnormally formed uteruses as shown by x-ray. Many of the uteruses were T-shaped (*see* illustrations, next page) as compared to the normal triangular shape, and many were smaller than normal (hypoplastic). He also noted shaggy and bumpy uterine linings compared to the normally smooth uterine lining. And he found constrictions around some of the uteruses and around the uterine horns, the junctions at which the uterus branches into each fallopian tube.

These findings have been confirmed by other doctors, including Dr. Merle Berger of Boston and Dr. Arthur Haney of Duke University.

## Reproductive Difficulties of DES Daughters

As DES daughters reach the age when they are most likely to bear children, it has become increasingly obvious that something is wrong. While there are disagreements in the medical community about the nature of the problems, the consensus is that DES daughters *do* in fact have more problems having babies than other women do. The problems include inability to conceive (primary infertility), repeated miscarriages, incompetent cervix (often the reason for the repeated miscarriages), ectopic, or tubal, pregnancy, and premature delivery resulting in stillbirths.

*Inability to conceive.* There seems to be a major difference of opinion among DES-knowledgeable physicians as to whether

# Normal uterus

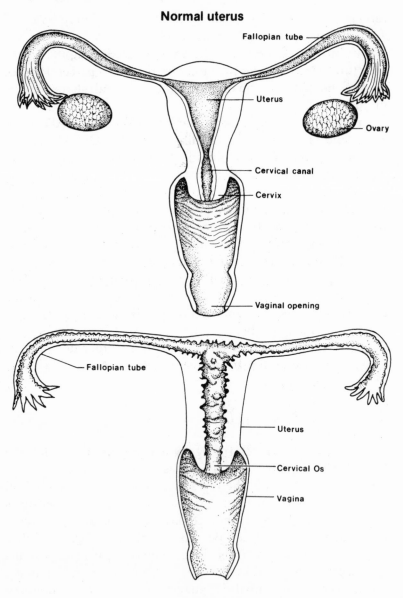

Fallopian tube

Uterus

Ovary

Cervical canal

Cervix

Vaginal opening

Fallopian tube

Uterus

Cervical Os

Vagina

## T-shaped uterus

or not DES daughters have more than average difficulty becoming pregnant. Some physicians, such as Dr. Ann Barnes (codirector of the DESAD project at the Massachusetts General Hospital) and Dr. Larry Cousins of the University of California at San Diego have found, in separate studies, that there appear to be no significant differences in ability to conceive between DES daughters and young women not exposed to DES.

By contrast, other doctors with equally good professional credentials *have* found a significantly higher incidence of infertility among DES daughters. One of these physicians, Dr. Arthur Herbst (director of the DES adenocarcinoma registry), compared 226 DES daughters with 203 control-group young women, both groups being part of the original Dieckmann study of 1953. Dr. Herbst found that twice as many DES daughters reported infertility. Interestingly, both Dr. Herbst and Dr. Barnes reported that at least 80 percent of the DES daughters in their respective studies eventually conceived and delivered live infants.

Two other Harvard physicians, Drs. Merle Berger and Donald Goldstein, studied 69 DES daughters and concluded that "DES-exposed women *do* have impaired reproductive function."

What these and other doctors have written about DES-related infertility problems is often at variance, so it is not surprising that the average physician in practice is confused, as are women themselves. The result is that many doctors in practice will believe what they want to believe and still be able to find enough scientific evidence to back up their opinions.

This can be a grave disservice to the DES daughter hoping to become pregnant. Consider Hannah, for example, whose story opens this chapter. When she asked her doctor, who is a prominent high-risk obstetrics specialist, about having a cerclage to avoid the possibility of losing her unborn child through an incompetent cervix, he told her that it was not necessary. One month later, Hannah miscarried because of an incompetent cervix. Had the DES experts writing about infertility and pregnancy problems in DES daughters been a little less blandly reassuring, perhaps Hannah's doctor would have reacted to her situation with a bit more caution by performing a preventive cerclage in time to save her pregnancy.

A good measure in deciding whether or not to take preventive measures, such as a cerclage, is the condition of a woman's cervix. If her cervix is malformed, the chances are there will also be upper genital tract malformations which may well make a pregnancy more difficult. A malformed cervix may also indicate a malformation of the cervical musculature, which might render it incompetent when the weight of the pregnant womb grows heavy enough to test it. Yet other DES daughters may miscarry because the musculature of their abnormally small uteruses is unable to stretch enough to accommodate the growing fetus.

*Why* DES daughters are having problems becoming pregnant is something else, and a number of reasons have been presented. One is that the DES-affected vaginal environment is poorly suited to the survival and movement of sperm. Two doctors from Cornell Medical College found that 75 percent of DES daughters in whom sperm motility (sperm movement) studies were done had such poor-quality vaginal and cervical mucus that the sperm had no medium in which to migrate through to the uterus and fallopian tubes. The doctors conjectured that this condition was due to DES-altered vaginal tissue which produced below-par mucus. They also found that DES daughters in the study had more fallopian tube defects than normal, which may have prevented the sperm from traveling upward to meet the ovum or the fertilized ovum from traveling back down to the uterus. The third problem they encountered was failure to ovulate.

Yet another suggestion has been that the shaggy, bumpy uterine lining found in many DES daughters makes an inhospitable surface for a fertilized ovum to implant itself in.

The result in any of these possible cases is primary infertility—inability to conceive.

*Repeated miscarriages and premature deliveries.* While doctors may argue about whether or not DES daughters are less fertile than other women, there is little disagreement about the unusually high number of miscarriages suffered by DES daughters once they do become pregnant. Universal medical experience indicates that, compared to other women, many more DES daughters have many more miscarriages during every stage of pregnancy.

Dr. Cousins of San Diego, who found no special difference between DES daughters and other women in their ability to conceive, *did* find that nearly half the pregnancies among DES daughters he studied ended prematurely (before the full 37 weeks of a normal-length pregnancy). For those daughters with gross abnormalities of the cervix and uterus, the percentage was even higher; more than 70 percent of pregnancies in this group ended in either miscarriage or in premature delivery and death of the fetus.

In his study of DES daughters and their unexposed counterparts born at the Chicago Lying-In Hospital during the DES study of 1952–53, Dr. Herbst reported findings similar to those of Dr. Cousins, namely, that the DES daughters had more miscarriages, more premature deliveries, and more stillborn babies.

Taken collectively, however, these studies indicate that most DES daughters, if they "keep trying," will eventually bear a live child.

*Cervical incompetence.* One of the more easily identifiable causes of miscarriage and premature delivery is an incompetent cervix, a cervix that dilates too soon during pregnancy, allowing the developing fetus to literally drop out of the uterus. According to several medical reports, DES daughters are subject to cervical incompetence more often than other women. Dr. Herbst's advice typifies that of other DES specialists. If an incompetent cervix is a possibility, more frequent examinations should be performed throughout pregnancy to check for early signs of dilation. If such signs are found, a cerclage may be performed. Shortly before the baby is due to be born, the stitches are removed. (Occasionally, the stitches are left in when a Caesarean birth is planned.)

One unusual case of cervical incompetence was reported from the University of Virginia School of Medicine. A DES daughter who underwent a cervical cerclage could not deliver her baby vaginally because her cervix refused to dilate following removal of the cerclage stitches, even after eight hours of normal labor. Her baby had to be delivered by Caesarean section. This case is simply another illustration of defective cervical musculature in DES daughters.

*Ectopic pregnancy.* One of the more serious pregnancy problems that seems to happen more often in DES daughters is tubal, or ectopic (outside the uterus), pregnancy.

Normally, sperm travel up through the uterus into the fallopian tube to fertilize the ovum. The fertilized egg then travels down the tube and into the uterus, where it soon implants and develops. An ectopic pregnancy is one in which the fertilized ovum implants and begins growing outside the uterus, often in the fallopian tube itself, a slim hollow reed of tissue that nature never intended for the expansion required by a developing embryo. The result can be life-threatening to the pregnant woman, if the tube ruptures and hemorrhages.

Tubal pregnancy requires speedy surgical intervention to remove the developing embryo, and to repair the tube, if possible, or to remove it if it is irreparably damaged.

Ectopic pregnancies are reported to occur in the general population in anywhere from one out of every 35 to one out of every 200 pregnancies. For DES daughters, the rate of such pregnancies is reported to occur *at least* five times as often, perhaps as frequently as one out of every *seven* pregnancies. Some doctors have speculated that this is due to an abnormal narrowing of the fallopian tubes where the tubes join the uterus, thus preventing the fertilized ovum from passing into the uterus.

## • DES DAUGHTERS AND CONTRACEPTION

The methods of contraception used by DES daughters and the popularity of each method closely parallel those used by their non-DES exposed counterparts. Among all young women studied, oral contraceptives (the Pill) are by far the most popular method of birth control. Over 65 percent of women report using the Pill, as compared to about 15 percent relying on intrauterine devices (IUDs), about 12 percent on diaphragms, and fewer than 8 percent of women depending on condoms and/or contraceptive foam.

Especially for DES daughters, the popularity of the Pill is somewhat unfortunate. While there is no hard evidence that the sex hormones contained in oral contraceptives can exacerbate the abnormalities present in DES daughters, more and more experts are advising that DES daughters NOT use them.

In its 1978 summary report, the government's DES Task Force wrote, "In view of the lack of information on long-term effects of estrogens in these women (DES daughters), the committee felt that oral contraceptives and other estrogens *should be avoided.*"

This opinion is shared by other physicians knowledgeable in the problems caused by DES. Dr. Stanley Robboy of the Massachusetts General Hospital in Boston and one of the pathologists for the Adenocarcinoma Registry reported an overgrowth of tiny glands in the adenosis tissue of DES daughters who used oral contraceptives. This glandular overgrowth has been termed by other doctors a relatively rare phenomenon, even in DES daughters. And, from the University of Chicago Dr. Herbst (as well as others) has advised his colleagues *not* to prescribe birth control pills for DES daughters.

One of the reasons for this recommendation is that no one knows if the cancer-causing effects of estrogens are cumulative, a possibility DES daughters were warned about in 1978 by Joseph Califano, former Secretary of the Department of Health, Education, and Welfare.

But even in the absence of hard evidence that DES daughters might be more susceptible to the cancer-causing potential of more estrogens, there is ample evidence that estrogen-containing oral contraceptives are capable of inducing tumor growth in *all* women, not merely in those exposed to DES. In 1977, Drs. Chan and Detmer of the University of Wisconsin reported benign liver tumors in long-term users of the Pill. And, much more recently, in a 1980 issue of the British medical journal *Lancet*, there was a report of malignant liver tumors resulting specifically from oral contraceptive use.

Even more thoroughly documented than liver tumors is the occurrence of endometrial cancer (cancer of the uterine lining) in young women who use estrogen-based oral contraceptives. Two physicians from the University of Washington reported in the March 6, 1980, issue of the *New England Journal of Medicine* that women who use estrogenic oral contraceptives run a nearly $7\frac{1}{2}$ times greater risk of developing endometrial cancer than nonusers. Of some comfort is that the incidence of endometrial cancer is lower in women who use oral contraceptives containing mostly progesterone-like hormones (synthetic progesterones) rather than estrogen.

DES Action, the consumer organization devoted solely to educating and informing people about DES, has published statements warning DES-exposed women *not* to use birth control pills.

"In our view," the editors of DES Action *Voice* write, "the evidence is against DES daughters using birth control pills that contain estrogen (almost all birth control pills contain estrogen). We would like to wait until the scientific community proves them safe before taking any more chances."

*Why you should avoid the "morning-after" birth control pill.* These same warnings apply to the DES morning-after pill. The rationale behind using DES as the so-called morning-after birth control pill is that high doses of estrogens taken shortly after intercourse cause abnormal changes, including edema (abnormal water retention) in the lining of the uterus. These changes create an inhospitable environment for the implantation of a fertilized egg. To be effective in preventing implantation, a woman must take two 25 milligram pills of DES per day for five consecutive days. In *Contraceptive Technology* 1978–1979, this dose is termed "a massive dose of synthetic estrogen," often causing nausea and vomiting. Other symptoms are headache, menstrual irregularities, and breast tenderness. About one out of every 200 women who take DES as a postcoital contraceptive will become pregnant despite treatment. Unless those pregnancies are aborted, the children born of them will have been exposed to massive doses of DES at the earliest and most vulnerable time of fetal development, producing more DES babies a full decade after DES was contraindicated for use in pregnant women.

Another very serious objection to the morning-after pill is that roughly eight out of every 10 women so treated are never pregnant in the first place, and so have been exposed to a dangerous drug for nothing! Barbara Seaman, coauthor of *Women and the Crisis in Sex Hormones*, reports that the morning-after birth control pill is especially popular on college campuses, where student health services dole it out with alarming nonchalance.

The message to DES daughters seems clear. While other methods of contraception may lack the convenience, the spontaneity, or the aesthetic appeal of the Pill, they may be far safer.

## Menstrual Irregularities

Scores of women who have written to DES Action for information have volunteered that they suffered from menstruation problems. But whether this problem is DES-related is, like so many other problems associated with DES exposure, a point of disagreement in the DES-knowledgeable medical community.

Dr. Ann Barnes of the Massachusetts General Hospital

DESAD Project is at one end of the spectrum. She has reported that no significant differences exist between the DES-
exposed and unexposed women in her clinical experience. At
the other end of the spectrum is Dr. Arthur Haney of Duke
University, who found that between 40 percent and 50 percent of his DES-exposed patients suffer some form of menstrual problem.

Somewhere between these two different experiences is Dr.
Herbst's finding, which shows that 10 percent of more than
200 DES daughters he studied had menstrual problems, as
compared to 4 percent of women in the control group.

The most commonly reported problems include infrequent
and scanty periods, dysmenorrhea (abnormally painful periods), and irregular periods. Dr. Grant Schmidt and co-workers
at the University of North Carolina found that one-third of
their DES-exposed patients who reported menstrual problems
did not ovulate. He also found that his patients' periods lasted
longer than those of nonexposed women.

To demonstrate once again how imprecise and incomplete
our knowledge still is about the effects of DES, there are
several other researchers who have found that the menstrual
periods of their DES-exposed patients are much *shorter* than
those of other women—lasting one to four days as contrasted
to the more usual five to eight days.

Although medical opinion is even more fragmented when it
comes to what to do about these problems, the chief value of
these reports to the DES daughter is that they will help her to
be taken more seriously by her physician when she does have
a problem.

## • THE PSYCHOLOGICAL IMPACT OF DES EXPOSURE

The most pervasive and yet perhaps the least well-defined
problem of DES-exposed offspring is the psychological one.

Fear, humiliation, anger, embarrassment, grief, and frustration are the unseen demons plaguing the DES daughter. As difficult as it is for adults to cope with these "demons," they take on even more ominous proportions when they beset the young adolescent DES daughter.

DES daughters are most likely to begin their extensive pelvic examinations at 12, 13, or 14. And, even under the best of circumstances, early adolescence is a time fraught with the pressures of growing up. As Dr. Serafina Corsello, a New York psychiatrist, reminded a group of more than 400 physicians at a DES seminar, adolescence is a time of "obsessional focusing" on the body. "The solitary pimple assumes the dimensions of an elephant's trunk. The sprouting of pelvic and axillary hair is often seen as an oddity. Their nose is too long, too short, too fat, too skinny and so on." In sum, she said, adolescents are in a stage of uneven development, and this unevenness awakens anxieties.

Of all the adjustments adolescents must make, emerging sexuality is the most threatening, according to Dr. Corsello.

What, then, is it like for a young girl barely emerging from childhood to undergo extensive and repeated examinations of her sex organs? There are differing opinions.

Some, like Fran Fishbane's, cofounder of DES Action and its former president, are pessimistic. Ms. Fishbane says, "I remain gloomy about the child going for her first examination. Can a young woman who has associated pain and anxiety with her vagina from the age of 12 then feel pleasure in that same area when she becomes sexually active years later?"

This question has been echoed by others who are concerned with the potentially devastating impact of early pelvic examinations. Those first examinations, others have cautioned, can set the tone for acceptance or denial of sexuality. Dr. Corsello warned that a bad medical experience could cause young girls to regard their sexual organs "as a source of pain, shame, and fear of death."

However, in spite of these grim warnings, there are many DES daughters who cope with their exposure without letting it destroy them. The mother of two teenaged DES daughters says that her daughters approach their pelvic examinations with less apprehension than they do their dental appointments.

What can be done to prevent emotional pain and scarring for young DES daughters? Part of the answer seems to lie in the daughter's relationship with her mother. If it is a good one, the daughter seems to be able to cope with the trauma of DES exposure far better than if she does not get along with her mother.

In the first scientific paper published about the psychological burdens of the DES-exposed, Dr. Ruth Schwartz and Nancy Stewart of the University of Rochester noted that daughters who were able to speak openly with their mothers were able to resolve their fears most effectively. Dr. Schwartz and Ms. Stewart recommended, though, that a preliminary session with a trained counselor before the first examination could be very helpful. Further, they stressed that *good physician-to-patient communication providing ample information at every stage of the examination is crucial to easing patient anxiety.*

The only other paper to date on the subject generally agreed with the Schwartz paper. Dr. Louis Burke and three colleagues from the Beth Israel Hospital in Boston titled their paper, "Observations on the Psychological Impact of Diethylstilbestrol Exposure and Suggestions on Management." These authors spoke at length about feelings of "resentment, disappointment, betrayal, anxiety, and helplessness" experienced by DES daughters and their mothers. They too suggested that physicians treat their DES-exposed patients with respect, that they acknowledge their patients' anxieties, and that they provide plenty of information. They also stressed that physicians offer their patients a well-structured plan for medical follow-up, and that they refer women to "support groups" for additional information and continued support.

*The impact of physician attitudes.* In spite of the good and helpful advice in the Burke paper, it is marred by a tone of medical condescension toward the woman patient. In discussing DES mothers, the authors describe "one of the best-integrated and happiest women we studied." Despite her initial fear and confusions, they wrote, this mother never allowed her DES exposure to threaten "her trust in physicians." Dr. Burke and his colleagues appear to be suggesting that unquestioning trust in doctors is somehow a requisite of good mental health!

These same authors concluded an otherwise good list of dos and don'ts for the physician by warning that an authoritarian approach to a patient may turn her "into a quietly rebellious, potential litigant." Although an angry patient *is* more likely to sue a doctor, one would hope that physicians would have more humanistic reasons for not being authoritarian.

Far worse than subtle underlying biases are the attempts by some DES-prescribing physicians to insure themselves immunity from lawsuits by destroying their patients' records. Rumors that many doctors have deliberately destroyed such documents have been borne out by scores of anecdotal reports. One DES daughter in Texas, for example, wrote that when she first called the doctor who delivered her, he was very glad to hear from her. But, upon hearing she wanted her mother's obstetrical records, he angrily denied prescribing DES and said that, besides, he had "lost" 10 years of his records.

There is no doubt that the utter failure of some doctors to communicate with their patients is the root of much anxiety. One 17-year-old DES daughter wrote that when she was 16 she sought birth control advice at a local clinic and was called back because a routine Pap smear indicated a premalignant condition. "It scared me so much," she wrote, "I just never went back to that clinic." It seems no one at the clinic took the time to explain to her what the findings meant in light of her DES exposure.

Yet another daughter wrote that she was "severely reprimanded for peeking" into her own medical file.

Dr. Charles Goodstein, a New York psychiatrist, says, "Despite so much lip service paid to the impact of psychological issues in medical practice, I'm afraid that a Neanderthal approach prevails ... in the examination ... of ... vulnerable young girls and women. I know many able and perceptive obstetricians, but so many never seem to notice women's faces. Can they be expected to recognize apprehension, despair, or low self-esteem? For many doctors, I'm sorry to say the answer is 'No.' "

## • PERSONALITY ALTERATIONS IN DES CHILDREN

Among the most elusive and yet most intriguing of the effects of DES have been the so-called "birth defects of the mind," permanent personality alterations alleged to occur in DES children as a result of their *in utero* exposure to the hormone.

June Machover Reinisch of Rutgers University studied the personalities and intelligence quotients of 75 children whose mothers had taken hormones during pregnancy. She reported that children exposed to progesterone-like hormones were significantly more self-assured, assertive, and independent than unexposed siblings, while children exposed *in utero* to estrogenic hormones, such as DES, were far less independent and self-sufficient.

Another researcher, Dr. Anke Ehrhardt, a psychiatry professor at Columbia University, compared the behavior of children between the ages of 8 and 14 whose mothers had taken either progesterone or estrogens (including DES). She concluded that girls so exposed appeared less "tomboyish" than unexposed girls of the same age. She also reported that boys exposed to female hormones prenatally appeared "less stereotypically masculine" than their unexposed peers. Dr. Ehrhardt suggested that her studies might indicate that only small amounts of female hormones are necessary to suppress the male hormones present during fetal development.

More recently, a fascinating paper on the alteration of brain chemistry from DES exposure adds credence to the work of Drs. Ehrhardt and Reinisch. Two researchers from the National Institute of Environmental Health Sciences found that the brain levels of norepinephrine (a substance closely related to adrenaline) were decreased in newborn male rats exposed to DES. The reduced levels of this chemical were similar to the lower levels normally found in female rats. The researchers concluded that DES administration had caused an "apparent feminization" in the brain chemistry of these immature rats and that this event might reflect brain chemistry development, "which becomes recognizable in the adult as sex-specific behavior." When you stop to consider that the level of development in newborn rats is analogous to a six- or seven-month-old human fetus, it becomes apparent that DES taken in pregnancy may well have affected the "sex-specific" behavior of human DES children.

Although the practical value of these studies seems vague, they nevertheless point up how little we know about the far-reaching effects of giving hormones (or, indeed, any drugs) to pregnant women.

## • HEALTH CARE RECOMMENDATIONS FOR DES DAUGHTERS

All DES daughters should have periodic gynecological examinations performed by a DES-knowledgeable physician. (For the names of physicians in your area qualified to examine a DES daughter, contact DES Action; see appendix for address.)

These examinations should begin at age 14 or after the first menstrual period, whichever comes first. Although the recommended frequency for these examinations varies, depending on which doctor you ask, the general rule is that DES daughters should be checked every six months to start with and, if all remains well, exams can generally be cut back to every 12 months when a woman reaches her twenties, which is after the incidence of clear-cell adenocarcinoma peaks.

Although some highly respected, DES-knowledgeable doctors are now advocating annual instead of semiannual examinations—even for younger, teenaged DES daughters—at least one case of clear-cell adenocarcinoma has been reported in a DES daughter who was receiving semiannual check-ups. When she reached 19, this DES daughter was found to have a just-beginning cancer, although prior exams had indicated all was normal. Based on this case, the reporting physician (Dr. B. Anderson of Tufts New England Medical Center) stressed the "necessity for frequent vaginal . . . examinations at intervals no greater than six months." In view of this case, it would seem wise to err in favor of caution and have semiannual check-ups. An extra exam per year is a small price to pay for peace of mind.

Expect the following procedures of a thorough DES pelvic examination.

1. *A fastidious palpation* of the entire vaginal and cervical surface. Your doctor will be checking for small lumps and irregularities frequently found in DES daughters. Remember, the chances are *overwhelmingly* in your favor that these irregularities are benign.

2. *A Pap (Papanicolaou) smear* will be taken with samples from several locations around the cervix and the vagina. This is the same test used for every woman who has a yearly pelvic examination. (Doctors refer to it as a cytologic exam.)

*3. *Schiller's (or Lugol's) iodine test*. In this procedure, which was commonly used before the development of the Pap smear, the cervix and vaginal walls are coated with a solution of iodine. Abnormal tissue, including adenosis, immature metaplasia,

---

*There is some difference of medical opinion about the need for both the Schiller's test and colposcopy since they have some overlapping functions. However, if your physician does not have a colposcope, medical authorities strongly recommend the iodine test.

dysplasia, carcinoma *in situ*, and clear-cell adenocarcinoma, will not stain the characteristic brown color that the surrounding normal tissue stains. It is important to remember that any irregularities revealed by this test, as with the palpation, are virtually always benign.

Dr. Eugene Sandburg of the Stanford University School of Medicine writes that "infinitesimally little" of what fails to stain is cancer. The value of the iodine test is that it serves to highlight irregular tissue, making it easier to observe. The application of the iodine solution may cause a mild stinging or burning sensation in some women.

*4. *Colposcopy*. The colposcope looks something like elaborate binoculars on a swinging arm attached to the wall or to a floor stand. Viewing the cervix and vagina through the colposcope, the physician can examine these tissues with the benefit of magnification. Another advantage of the colposcope is that photographs of cervical and vaginal abnormalities can be taken, providing a permanent visual record. Because direct visualization is possible through the colposcope, it is also an extremely helpful tool in locating abnormal tissue, which has been identified by Pap smear as requiring a biopsy.

5. *Biopsy*. If your Pap smear examination reveals abnormal cells, your doctor may biopsy the suspicious areas. This consists of snipping small bits of tissue, which are then sent to a pathologist for microscopic examination. These biopsies are performed in the doctor's office and although there is some discomfort, the procedure generally doesn't require anesthesia. The exception to this might be in very young girls.

### • WHAT IF YOU HAVE A CONDITION THAT REQUIRES TREATMENT?

Three conditions definitely require treatment: dysplasia, carcinoma *in situ*, and clear-cell adenocarcinoma. Although dysplasia, per se, is not cancerous, it will—in a significant number of cases—progress to carcinoma *in situ* and then to invasive cancer, according to Dr. Leopold Koss of the Albert Einstein College of Medicine. Although dysplasia and carcinoma *in situ*, which are similar, may disappear spontaneously in some cases even after a simple biopsy, prudence dictates that these conditions be treated more thoroughly. The following, briefly described treatments are the ones most frequently used.

*Conization.* This is a small surgical procedure whereby a cone-shaped piece of tissue is removed with the widest end containing the dysplasia or carcinoma *in situ* on the cervical or vaginal surface. The cut margins are then stitched together. Although this is a commonly performed procedure, there are several disadvantages for the patient. First, it requires hospitalization and anesthesia, often a general anesthetic. Second, the healing period may be longer than with other treatments. Third, there is considerable debate about whether cervical conization adversely affects a woman's ability to subsequently become pregnant, and/or to maintain the pregnancy.

*Cryosurgery.* This procedure involves the destruction of tissue through the application of extreme cold, usually supercooled gas applied with a special probe.

This method has achieved wide popularity for treating such conditions as cervical intra-epithelial neoplasia, dysplasia, and carcinoma *in situ*. The advantages of this treatment over surgery are that it can be performed in a doctor's office, requires no anesthesia, and allows complete healing within four months. After two weeks the woman is sufficiently healed to allow sexual intercourse.

General disadvantages of cryosurgery are that it causes a heavy, watery discharge for the first two weeks following the procedure, and can cause moderate discomfort during the procedure.

However, *DES daughters should be forewarned that cryosurgery may well cause chronic problems for them.* Dr. Grant Schmidt of the University of North Carolina found that 75 percent of DES daughters treated with cryosurgery for cervical lesions developed stenosis, or blockage, of the cervical canal, compared to fewer than 1 percent of DES-unexposed women. Dr. Schmidt and his co-investigator, Dr. W. Fowler, warn that this may indicate an abnormal healing response in DES daughters. "Locally destructive methods such as cryosurgery, cauterization (burning), and excision (conization) have resulted in permanent and significant physical damage [in DES daughters]."

*Laser treatment.* Laser treatment, the newest therapy for treating noninvasive cervical and vaginal lesions may well be the least damaging for DES daughters. The treatment, called $CO_2$ laser tissue evaporation, was first used to treat gynecological lesions in Birmingham, England, in 1977.

Its advantages are that it requires no anesthesia, with the majority of patients reporting no discomfort whatever during treatment, no posttreatment bleeding in the great majority of patients, and little or no vaginal discharge. Complete healing takes place within six weeks, and there is little or no scarring. The laser beam, no wider than a pencil line, can be precisely controlled both in width and depth, so that no normal tissue is destroyed.

Dr. Burton Krumholz, associate chairman of the Department of Obstetrics and Gynecology at the Long Island Jewish-Hillside Medical Center in New York, is enthusiastic about the advantages of laser therapy for DES daughters, but cautions that it should be performed *only* by a doctor experienced in the technique who is also an expert in colposcopy. However, because it is relatively new, this treatment is not yet widely available.

*Treatment for clear-cell adenocarcinoma.* The treatment of choice for vaginal clear-cell adenocarcinoma is radical surgery. This means removal of the vagina, the cervix, uterus, fallopian tubes, and some lymph glands. Often, if the cancer is an early one, the ovaries are left intact so that the woman does not experience premature menopause.

This treatment is drastic, but experience has shown that DES daughters who have had only local excision of even very small tumors tend to have a recurrence of cancer. (*See* chapter 3, page 40, for a discussion of survival and recurrence rates.) With radical surgery, the chances of complete recovery and cure approach 90 percent. Radiation has also been used both as primary treatment and in conjunction with surgery, but many physicians are reluctant to expose young women to the long-range hazards of high doses of radiation. So, surgery remains the treatment of choice.

*Vaginal reconstruction.* Because DES daughters who develop cancer are very young, with virtually their entire adult (and sexually active) lives ahead of them, most surgeons perform immediate vaginal reconstruction (as soon as they remove the cancerous vagina). However, there is still a great deal of uncertainty about the best method for vaginal reconstruction.

Although a number of vagina "substitutes" have been used to surgically recreate an absent vagina, the use of a section of the patient's own skin to create a vagina seems to be the most effective and least traumatic reconstructive technique. The skin graft may be applied immediately following the vaginectomy or seven to ten days later. A large tamponlike piece of foam rubber covered by a condom is inserted to maintain the shape of the graft until new tissue has a chance to regenerate and grow around the graft. One doctor who performed this procedure on a 19-year-old DES daughter reported that the woman was "sexually active and orgasmic" four months after her operation!

Other, less successful techniques have included removing a section of the large intestine and then sewing it in place as a neo-vagina. This technique has many drawbacks, not the least of which is that it subjects the woman to gastrointestinal surgery which, in turn, can create urinary incontinence lasting as long as six months. In addition, an intestinal or colon neo-vagina produces quantities of mucus, causing substantial personal hygiene problems.

A new technique for vaginal reconstruction using a special kind of skin flap has also been tried. These "flaps," called myocutaneous skin flaps, involve transferring sections of skin and underlying muscle—often from the inner thigh—and swinging these sections into place as neo-vaginas. Because these flaps are not completely severed from the thigh, their original blood supplies remain intact and the graft retains its viability. However, some patients undergoing this procedure have complained of painful and sometimes debilitating thigh scars.

## A Final Word

Although most DES-affected people—mothers and sons, as well as daughters—are frightened and upset upon first learning of the hazards of their exposure, it is important to remember that with proper health care and regular examinations the chances are excellent that they will live normal and healthy lives.

# 5·The Sons of DES

*"Why is it so hard to get DES sons to come forward? The fact is that men do not easily talk about genital problems. . . . In our society the stigma attached to genital problems totally threatens the male identity. If a man is impotent or sterile, he is made to feel less of a man."*

A DES son, DES Action **Voice,** *Vol. 2, No. 1*

Yet another irony of the DES fiasco is that the whole, nasty business has been labeled "a women's problem," a myth widely shared by men and women alike. But, the *fact* is that the unhappy legacy of DES is definitely *not* for women only.

According to the most reliable estimates to date, about one-third of the one to one and one-half million DES sons in the United States have a physical problem because they were exposed to DES before they were born. That's half a million American boys and men.

But in spite of their huge numbers, they might well be called "the hidden half-million," hidden because few people, including doctors, mothers, and the sons themselves, are aware that DES sons *do* have problems. There are a number of reasons for this. For one thing, as far as is known now, DES sons—unlike daughters—do *not* get cancer as a direct result of their prenatal exposure to the drug. Second, far fewer sons than daughters seem to have DES-related abnormalities, re-sulting in fewer scientific studies of male problems. And finally, as the quote above suggests, men in our society (in contrast to women) just don't talk about their own genital problems because such problems are considered to be a threat to the man's fundamental sense of maleness.

The collective result is that practically no information at all about DES sons has percolated through to the public. This is misleading.

The most dependable scientific studies have shown that three out of every 10 DES sons have one or more DES-related problems of the urogenital tract. These run the gamut from harmless and painless to grossly malfunctional. They range from cysts inside the scrotal sacs that can be felt but that cause no problems, to malformations of the penis, to sterility.

Most of the following information comes from published studies done at the University of Chicago by Dr. William Gill, a urologist, and Dr. Marluce Bibbo, a gynecologist-obstetrician, and their colleagues. The University of Chicago team is one of the few groups in the country investigating in depth the problems of DES sons. The population base for these studies is the same children born of the women included in the original 1951–1952 Dieckmann study described in chapter 2. While Dr. Dieckmann perhaps never intended that his study be expanded to cover the entire lifetimes of the DES babies involved, he designed it so well, including matched controls for every DES-exposed baby, that this Chicago population is an ideal one to observe. In addition, Dr. Dieckmann was far-sighted enough to computerize his data, which means that information can be retrieved, factors compared, and new information stored far more accurately than would be the case without computers.

The abnormalities I describe below have been well-documented in the University of Chicago DES sons and have been corroborated by other, smaller studies.

## • BENIGN ABNORMALITIES IN DES SONS

*Epididymal cysts.* Among the most frequently found abnormalities in DES sons are cysts in the epididymis, a long, thin, coiled tube which is continuous with the testicles and is also housed in the scrotal sacs (*see* illustration). In the mature male, sperm are manufactured in the testicles and then travel into the epididymis, where they reside and mature for about two weeks before they can be ejaculated. During this maturation process, the sperm acquire the ability to move (motility), which is one of the key qualities necessary for fertilizing an ovum. If a man's sperm have little or no ability to move, the man will be sterile.

For reasons still not understood, DES sons have an unusually high number of cysts in the epididymis. These cysts appear to be harmless and need not be treated unless they are uncomfortable. They are generally filled with a clear, straw-colored fluid which does not contain sperm. Epididymal cysts occur in more than two out of every ten DES sons. Although some doctors have estimated that one out of every twenty men *not* exposed to DES have these cysts, they are uncommon enough that many urologists have never seen even one! For example, Dr. David Uehling, a professor of urology at the University of Wisconsin Medical School who has been in practice for more than 20 years says he has never come across a single patient with such a cyst.

*Hypospadias.* The external genitalia of both sexes are formed from the same early embryonic tissue. In the female, this tissue gives rise to the vaginal labia; in the male, these folds of tissue fuse lengthwise into a hollow shaft to form the penis. Hypospadias is the name given to the condition in which the fusion is either incomplete or has not taken place at all.

To explain further, imagine a section of garden hose with a seam down the length of it. Now imagine that during the manufacture of that hose, the seam was imperfectly sealed so that openings remain along the side of the hose through which water can spurt out. In hypospadias, urine comes out of an opening along the side of the penis rather than from the tip. Hypospadias can occur at any point along the length of the penis. At least one doctor who studied nine DES sons with hypospadias found that the distance between the hypospadias opening and the base of the penis correlated well with the precise week during pregnancy that each of their mothers began taking synthetic hormones.

But, hypospadias does not occur *only* in boys whose mothers took hormones during pregnancy. About one out of every 700 boys born to all women has the condition. Although there are no estimates for how much more often hypospadias occurs in DES sons than in boys *not* exposed to hormones, the Chicago studies do indicate the condition occurs significantly more often in the DES-exposed.

*Microphallus.* An abnormally small penis (microphallus) is another condition that occurs with significant frequency in DES sons. In a recent study of 308 sons, the University of Chicago researchers found four men with microphallus, compared to none in the DES-*un*exposed group. Locker room jokes about small penises notwithstanding, a penis is judged to be microphallic only if it is shorter than 4 centimeters while flaccid. As is to be expected, such a small penis is not sexually adequate.

*Indurations and varicoceles of the testicles.* Other less common but still distinct abnormalities affecting DES sons include indurations and varicoceles of the testicles.

An induration is a thickening such as might be formed by scar tissue; this can be felt upon palpation. Testicular calcifications have also been reported to occur more often in DES sons; these are lumps within the testicle, which can be distinguished from indurations by their rock-hardness.

A testicular varicocele is an abnormally swollen or varicose vein of the testicle. Varicoceles also seem to occur more often in DES sons, and even more often yet, in DES sons with unusually small testicles. Varicoceles are surgically correctable.

*Urethral strictures and other urinary tract abnormalities.* When doctors at the University of Southern California sent questionnaires to the mothers of DES sons, 300 responded, along with a similar number of mothers who did not take DES. The answers these women gave indicated that the DES sons, in contrast to the nonexposed sons, had significantly more problems of the urogenital tract. These problems included infections, trouble passing urine due either to strictures of the urethra or to hypospadias, kidney and bladder pain, and penile bleeding and other abnormal discharges.

Unfortunately, the DES sons in this survey were not examined by the physicians conducting the study, and so the information given by the mothers could not be confirmed directly.

*Sperm and semen abnormalities.* Sperm abnormalities may indicate something wrong with the quality of the sperm, the quantity, or with both.

Normal sperm concentration, or quantity, is about 60 million sperm per milliliter of ejaculate, with a count lower than 20 million sperm per milliliter considered sub- or in-fertile, although there are cases on record of men with sperm counts of 10 million having fathered children.

The quality of sperm is generally measured by a grading system called the Eliasson method or MacCleod's criteria. A sperm sample is given a score from one to 10 based on four factors: sperm concentration, the relative number of motile sperm, the vigor with which the sperm move, and the percentage of sperm with an abnormal shape. The higher the Eliasson score, the more abnormal the sperm sample. A collective grade of less than 1 is considered normal; 2 to 4 is doubtful; 5 to 10 is pathological; and greater than 10 is considered severely pathological.

A normal sperm consists of an oval-shaped head, a "neck," and a long tail. Abnormal sperm forms manifest themselves variously—with double heads or double tails, with abnormally small heads, irregularly shaped heads, short or almost absent tails, and other oddities. These sperm are incapable of fertilizing an ovum.

Nearly one-quarter of DES sons examined at the University of Chicago had an Eliasson score of 10 or more, and nearly 40 percent had a score greater than 5. These figures are in stark contrast to those from the control group, where only 3 percent of men had severely pathological sperm, and only 14 percent had Eliasson scores of greater than 5.

The men examined in this study were in their mid- to late twenties when examined, an age when most have not yet begun to try fathering children. But, according to their predictive Eliasson scores, well over one-third may never be able to father children. And, according to a new technique for determining male fertility, this number may yet prove to be higher (*see* section in this chapter on the Sperm Penetration Assay, page 91).

More DES sons than their unexposed counterparts also had abnormalities of semen, the sticky, whitish fluid medium in which sperm is ejaculated. DES sons had a somewhat lower total ejaculate volume than normal and their semen samples did not clot properly—a factor that could adversely affect sperm motility.

*Undescended and hypoplastic testicles.* From the point of view of a cancer threat, by far the most serious of DES-related abnormalities in sons are undescended testicles and hypoplastic (unusually small) testicles. It is well established that both abnormalities are associated with an increased risk of testicular cancer.

Although the testicles are basically formed before the second month of fetal life, they do not descend into the scrotal sacs (where they then remain for the life of the male), until the eighth month of fetal life. Between fetal months two and eight, the testicles grow and mature inside the abdominal cavity.

Occasionally, one of the testicles will remain in the abdominal cavity even after birth. This is called an undescended testicle. When this happens, the affected testicle is usually sterile, perhaps due to the higher temperature inside the body or to some basic developmental flaw. Only rarely do both testicles in the same individual remain undescended. Most undescended testicles are also abnormally small, although not all hypoplastic testicles had problems descending.

Whatever prenatal influence causes a testicle to be abnormally small or to remain undescended also seems to predispose it to developing cancer. This is true for *all* men with the problem, not just for DES sons. But, because DES sons have a much higher incidence of undescended and hypoplastic testicles than other men, their chances for developing testicular cancer are also that much greater.

At one time, doctors advised surgically lowering an undescended testicle into the scrotum well before a boy reached puberty. Now, however, it is well recognized that because this procedure does *not* diminish that testicle's higher risk for developing a malignancy, surgical removal of the undescended testicle is preferable.

Twenty-six of 308 DES sons from the Chicago study as compared to only six of 301 men from the control group had hypoplastic or undescended testicles. Twenty-one of these 26 men—a walloping 80 percent—had pathologic or severely pathologic sperm samples as measured by the Eliasson method, even with one testicle that was presumably normal.

### • THE FETAL DEVELOPMENT OF THE MALE GENITALIA

The initial development of the male genitalia takes place before the seventh week of fetal life, generally before most women began taking DES. Although the initial formation of the male genitals may have escaped being affected by DES, subsequent growth and development *were* taking place during exposure.

This may help to explain such errors in growth and development as microphallus and undescended testicles.

In contrast, the female genitalia are not completely formed until the twentieth week of fetal life—long after most mothers began taking DES. The probability that initial male genital formation was complete before most mothers began taking DES may help account for the fact that far fewer DES sons have structural abnormalities than do DES daughters.

# • THE RISKS OF DES-RELATED CANCERS IN SONS

Exposure to DES *following* initial genital formation may also help to explain why there is no known direct relationship between prenatal DES exposure and cancer in sons, such as there is in daughters.

However, there is a well-established *indirect* relationship, as I have already mentioned between undescended and hypoplastic testicles and cancer, even if undescended testicles are surgically placed in the scrotum. Some doctors estimate that these abnormal testicles have at least a 10 times higher risk of developing cancer, while others have estimated that the risk might be as high as 1,000-fold greater. (I should mention here that testicular cancer accounts for about 2 percent of all cancers affecting males at any age and affects roughly four out of every 100 white males in the United States, but since the disease occurs mainly in men between the ages of 25 and 32 years, the incidence for testicular cancer is higher for this age group.) This increased risk for developing cancer is the same *whether or not* the individual has a history of prenatal hormone exposure. Theoretically, then, DES sons with their higher incidence of testicular maldescent should also have a higher incidence of testicular cancer. I caution the reader, however, that no such increased risk has yet been demonstrated.

For DES sons whose testicles are normal, there is no known increase in the risk of testicular cancer. However, a preliminary report by Dr. Stanley Robboy (one of the pathologists working with the DES cancer registry) and two other physicians did indicate that there might indeed be an increased risk. To translate from the cautious language of medical scientists, while there is no *hard evidence* that DES sons with undescended testicles are developing more testicular cancer than others, it sure looks like they are. But, just to point up the many unknowns and oddities doctors are finding in trying to determine the precise risk for DES-associated testicle cancer, Dr.

Robboy and his associates also reported that all men who wear briefs as opposed to boxer shorts have a three times higher risk for developing testicle cancer!

Like DES daughters, DES sons are still relatively young, and no one can be sure what will happen as these men age. But still, predictions are made, and like most other theories, they can be confusing and contradictory. At least some scientists have predicted that, as they enter their fifties and sixties, DES sons will be beset by more prostate cancer than other men. The basis for this theory lies in the fact that the prostate gland has the same embryonic tissue origin as the vagina which, of course, is the site of DES-related cancer in women.

Will prostatic tissue sensitized decades earlier by prenatal exposure to DES be ultrasensitive to the carcinogenic effects of the aging process? Dr. William Gill says, "I am optimistic in nature, but there is really no evidence to predict one way or the other on prostatic cancer incidence and tumor behavior in these men exposed to DES in utero."

Ironically, DES is among the most popular chemotherapeutic treatments currently available for advanced prostate cancer. This malignancy is dependent upon the male hormone, androgen. When DES is administered, it seems to have a counteractive effect on the hormone-sensitive tissue of the tumor, and the tumor often shrinks. DES is not a cure for prostate cancer, but it can significantly decrease pain and improve the quality of life for men treated with it. But, there is a catch even in these apparently successful results. Men treated with DES for prostate cancer run a higher than normal risk of developing breast cancer!

Dr. David Rose, an expert in the relationship of hormones and the development of cancer, conjectures that male breast tissue—unaccustomed to even small amounts of estrogen—is super-sensitive to the carcinogenic potential of even moderate daily doses of an estrogenic chemical such as DES. (The daily doses of DES to treat prostate cancer usually range from 2 to 5 milligrams, less than one-fiftieth the daily dose many pregnant women received.) Whether Dr. Rose's conjecture is correct or whether other factors are involved, one thing seems sure: Where hormone treatments are concerned, there are no free rides.

That hormone treatments, specifically DES treatments, could backfire and cause abnormalities and cancer has been shown by many investigators in studies as early as 1938 and continuing to the present. But, perhaps the most unsettling paper of all is one that was written 40 years ago, the same year that the Food and Drug Administration approved DES for clinical use. The paper describes nearly every DES-related abnormality we are now seeing in human males.

The authors of the paper, three doctors from Northwestern University, detailed the results of feeding DES to pregnant mice. Drs. Greene, Burrill, and Ivy wrote that virtually all the male offspring of the DES-dosed pregnant mice suffered genital anomalies. These included undescended and hypoplastic testicles, hypospadias, microphallus, and epididymal hypoplasia. Somehow, neither the Smiths, who proposed DES to treat pregnant women, nor the drug companies that produced and profited from DES heeded this work or considered it relevant to humans. The authors were so clear and thorough in cataloging the DES-caused abnormalities they found, it seems impossible that they could have been so completely ignored for so long.

### • THE SPERM PENETRATION ASSAY AND DES SONS

The possibilities for cancer and benign abnormalities notwithstanding, the real blight on the lives of many DES sons may yet prove to be infertility. According to a new test for male infertility—a test which, as of this writing (November 1980), is barely beyond the experimental stage and not widely available—a much higher percentage of DES sons than was previously believed may be unable to father children.

Called the sperm penetration assay, or SPA for short, the new test was first applied to DES sons by Dr. Morton Stenchever, chairman of the Department of Obstetrics and Gynecology at the University of Washington in Seattle. Briefly, the test consists of taking a sample of ejaculated human semen and incubating it with specially prepared hamster eggs. If fewer than 15 percent of the hamster eggs have been penetrated by the sperm after two hours of incubation, the man is judged infertile.

Developed by Dr. Ryuzo Yanamaguchi of the University of Hawaii Medical School, the SPA permits the occurrence of a phenomenon in laboratory test tubes that does not happen in nature, namely, the penetration of eggs from one species by the sperm from another species. To accomplish this, Dr. Yanamaguchi devised a technique for stripping the eggs of their protective coating following their removal from the hamster. The protective coating would otherwise prevent penetration by an alien sperm.

The assay, according to Dr. Stenchever, is close to 100 percent accurate. Compare this to the 70 percent accuracy rate of the standard laboratory measures of fertility and the SPA is impressive indeed. The Eliasson method or MacCleod's criteria may inaccurately determine the fertility or sterility of as many as three out of every ten men. In other words, a man whose Eliasson rating indicates normal fertility could, in fact, be unable to father a child, and conversely, a man whose sperm count and motility are judged subfertile by the Eliasson method may go on to pass the "ultimate" fertility test by eventually fathering a child.

The SPA appears to be a more accurate gauge because it gets at the heart of male fertility: the sperm's ability to penetrate an ovum. The Eliasson method, on the other hand, measures only related characteristics such as numbers of sperm and their ability to move. A semen sample may appear absolutely normal according to these fertility-related qualities, but the sperm may still, for reasons unknown, lack the ability to penetrate—and thus fertilize—an ovum. It is this final measure of fertility that the SPA reveals.

In applying the SPA to the diagnosis of human infertility,

Dr. B. Jane Rogers, also of the University of Hawaii, found the test nearly foolproof. Forty of the 44 men judged infertile by the SPA in actuality were unable to father children; the remaining four have not yet tried to father a child, but are presumed infertile. The sperm samples from these men fertilized fewer than 14 percent of the test hamster eggs, whereas anywhere from 15 percent to 100 percent of the hamster eggs were penetrated by sperm when mixed with the semen samples of men from the group presumed to be fertile. Neither sperm counts of above 10 million sperm per milliliter nor degree of sperm motility seemed to correlate with the SPA results.

Dr. Stenchever and his team of fertility specialists applied the SPA to DES sons almost by accident. In testing and refining the technique, they sought a group of men who might potentially have infertility problems but who were still young enough not to have tried to father children. DES sons fit the bill. The results, Dr. Stenchever told me, were decidedly *not* what he had expected.

Thirteen DES sons and 11 men not exposed to DES volunteered for Dr. Stenchever's study. The men ranged in age from 17 years to their late thirties. None of the volunteers—either from the DES group or from the control group—had any reason to believe he had a fertility problem. Semen samples from the volunteers were first tested by conventional fertility measures; all 24 volunteers were judged fertile. But, when portions of these same semen samples were subjected to the SPA, an astounding 10 of the 13 DES sons were judged infertile as compared to only one man from the control group.

"I was not prepared for the results we got," Dr. Stenchever told me in a telephone interview. However, he cautioned against overreacting to the results. The number of men in his study, he pointed out, is very small. And at least two cases of infertility in his DES volunteers were apparently reversed following surgery to correct varicoceles.

Still, the Stenchever findings are startling enough to warrant a much larger investigation. Based on his preliminary results, Dr. Stenchever has applied for funding to study many more DES sons with the SPA. If future findings bear out the results of this early study, it will mean that DES sons have inherited as unhappy a legacy as their DES sisters.

The Stenchever findings merely accentuate the most bitter DES irony of all. That is, the drug given to women to promote fertility may prevent fertility a generation later in the very "babies" it was intended to save.

## • WHAT TO DO IF YOU ARE A DES SON

If you are a DES son, the cautionary steps you should take are relatively simple and should *not* alarm you.

First, if you have not yet done so, get yourself examined by a urologist, a physician who specializes in problems of the male urogenital tract. Preferably, the urologist should be one who is familiar with DES-related problems. (For help in finding a doctor, contact DES Action or your local medical society; *see* appendix.)

The examination you receive will consist basically of two parts, a thorough physical examination and a laboratory check of your urine and semen. Your doctor should also take your complete medical history, including problems you may have had, and at what point during pregnancy and for how long your mother took DES.

The physical examination should include a visual inspection of your genitals to check for abnormalities, a thorough palpation of your scrotal sacs to check your testicles and epididymis for irregularities, and a prostate check. Many men find the prostate examination the most uncomfortable part of the physical, not because it is painful (it is *not* painful), but because it is awkward. To briefly describe a prostate exam, the doctor gently inserts a gloved, lubricated index finger into the rectum; it is through the rectal wall that the prostate gland can be palpated. A healthy prostate gland feels firm and well-defined, but soft; a cancerous prostate may have nodules or it may be rock-hard.

Although a number of blood tests have been developed in recent years designed to detect prostate cancer by measuring abnormal amounts of enzymes, the most recent reviews still cite the digital rectal (finger in the rectum) examination as the fastest, least expensive, and most widely available test for prostate cancer. And, according to a review in the August 28, 1980, issue of the *New England Journal of Medicine,* it is also highly accurate. Although I am not aware of an official recommendation regarding how often a DES son should have a prostate examination, it seems prudent for DES sons to have a digital rectal prostate check as a routine part of a yearly physical. I say this bearing in mind that the prostate is formed from the same embryonic tissue as the vagina, that the vagina is the site of DES-caused cancer in the daughters, and that the incidence of prostate cancer increases significantly in the entire male population as men grow older. Although you may find the digital rectal examination uncomfortable and embarrassing, remember it is quick, painless, and cheap insurance against a treatable condition developing into untreatable cancer. Keep in mind, though, that *so far* there is *no* evidence that DES sons have any more prostate problems than other men.

*Laboratory tests.* A sample of your urine will be examined for signs of infection (red blood cells, white blood cells or pus, bacteria), and for kidney malfunctions (albumin in the urine, excessive protein, and so on).

To provide a semen sample for laboratory analysis, you must masturbate to climax and ejaculate into a clean dish your doctor will provide for you. Every man I have spoken with who has undergone this procedure has reported feeling embarrassed and ill-at-ease having to masturbate on "command" and in the sterile environment of the doctor's office. In addition, some men may have religious prohibitions against masturbating. In this case, the DES son may be able to obtain special religious dispensation for medical purposes, or his

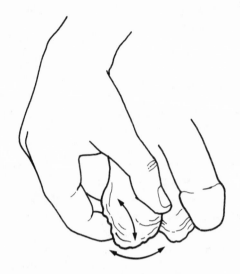

**Examine each testicle
with a gentle rolling action.**

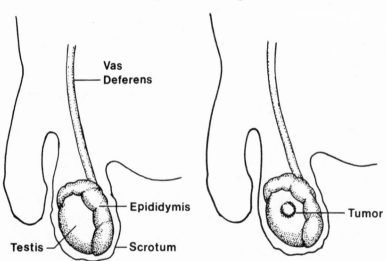

doctor may provide him with a special condom to use during regular intercourse; this special condom can collect and preserve for a short time a semen sample for subsequent analysis.

Remember that whatever your feelings about this part of the examination, a semen analysis is an integral part of your medical evaluation as a DES son, that your doctor will treat you with dignity, and that you will be given complete privacy. If your semen analysis is less than optimal, there may be treatments available (such as surgical correction for varicoceles), which can correct the abnormality.

*Testicular self-examination.* Chances are your doctor will conclude your examination with instructions to perform monthly testicular self-examinations. Because cancer of the testicles is a young man's disease, a monthly check of your own testicles should become a routine good health habit, just as monthly breast self-examination is for women.

The examination takes only a minute. Doctors recommend that you examine your testicles either in the shower or right after a shower because the skin of the scrotal sacs will be more relaxed. To examine yourself, simply roll each testicle gently between the fingers of both your hands. Feel for any irregularity, bump, or hardening. (*See* illustrations.)

If you should find something suspicious, don't panic. *Do* have your doctor check it. Remember—chances are good it is *not* cancer.

For additional information, the names of support groups in your area, and for help in finding a physician, see the appendix.

# 6·DES Mothers

*"The 'blame-the-mother' undercurrents that I sense sometimes in articles about DES aggravate me for just this reason. They are just like the 'blame-the-victim' myths about rape."*

A DES daughter, DES Action **Voice,** *Vol. 1, No. 4*

Every disaster generates profound and long-lasting consequences. As a medical disaster, DES is no different. For the millions of DES sons and daughters, the impact is obvious: these children must cope for the rest of their lives with the drug's effects on their bodies.

For their mothers the consequences of having taken DES are less clear. No one has to tell these women about the anguish of discovering that they have been the instruments, however inadvertent, of ill health and sometimes death for their children. But what DES mothers *do* need to be told, and what they are *not* being told, is that the DES they took one, two, or three decades ago may well affect their own health.

## • CANCER AND DES MOTHERS

In the small, cluttered offices of women's groups, in the quiet of private living rooms, in passing chit-chat between nurses, stories have been told of an inordinately large number of DES mothers developing breast cancer.

Since 1971, when the DES cancer connection was made, the medical spotlight has been turned on daughters. Much less light has been shed on DES sons, and virtually none on mothers. None, that is, until a nurse working with the University of Chicago DES follow-up studies remarked to research physicians that she thought that many of the DES-exposed mothers in their study had died of breast cancer.

Because estrogens have long been associated with cancer in animals, the Chicago researchers decided to take a closer look at the mothers, although their study had not been originally intended to examine them.

The results of a preliminary check revealed that nine of the DES mothers had developed breast cancer in the 23 years since the DES study had been initiated, compared to only one mother in the control group. This was indeed alarming and sufficient evidence to undertake a more thorough study.

Over the next one and one-half years, the Chicago researchers surveyed 693 of the DES mothers and 668 of their control group mothers. The two groups of women were closely matched for such factors as numbers of pregnancies, age at first menstruation, family history of breast cancer, and use of oral contraceptives—all factors known to affect a woman's risk for developing breast cancer.

The study was titled "A Twenty-Five Year Follow-Up Study of Women Exposed to Diethylstilbestrol During Pregnancy," and it was published in the *New England Journal of Medicine* in April 1978. It reported that 32 DES mothers developed breast cancer compared to 21 control group mothers. Overall, 66 DES mothers developed some form of cancer compared to 46 control group mothers. In other words, nearly half again as many DES mothers as control group mothers developed some form of cancer, with breast cancer being the single, most frequently occurring type.

Although the authors (Drs. Marluce Bibbo, Arthur Herbst, and others) acknowledged that "we have the problem of explaining the excess" of cancers, especially of the breast, they found that the observed differences were *not* "statistically significant."* In other words, after analyzing the data with statistical methodology, they concluded that the differences in the number of cancers between the two groups could be due to chance alone. Although the authors added a note of caution about "continued surveillance" of DES mothers, many in the medical community read the Bibbo-Herbst report and heaved a collective sigh of relief. Many doctors were relieved, but not all.

One doctor publicly disputed the conclusions of the University of Chicago group. This single physician, Dr. Sidney M. Wolfe, director of Ralph Nader's Health Research Group, wrote to then Secretary of the Department of Health, Education, and Welfare Joseph Califano that "there is preliminary evidence ... of a substantial increase in breast cancer and other hormone-related cancer in women who were given DES" at the University of Chicago. Dr. Wolfe based his statements on a progress report filed with the National Institutes of Health by the Chicago researchers seven months prior to the publication of their paper in the *New England Journal of Medicine*.

In recounting the Chicago data to Secretary Califano, Dr. Wolfe did his own statistical analysis of the Chicago data. Unlike Bibbo, Herbst, and their colleagues, he concluded that the University of Chicago's DES mothers had a *significantly higher* incidence of breast and other hormone-related cancers (ovaries, cervix, and uterus) than their counterparts in the control group.

How could two groups—both unquestionably reputable— arrive at opposite conclusions by analyzing the same data?

---

*Significance—In statistical terms, the degree of probability that a finding results from factors *other* than chance occurrence, and is expressed as a "p" value ("p" for probability). A finding is judged *not* due to chance alone if the p value is less than, commonly, 5 percent (.05), although the significant p value may differ according to individual circumstances. To explain further, if the findings in a given situation have a p value of .05 or less, this means that there is a 5 percent or less chance that the results are due to chance alone. Such findings are then judged to be "statistically significant."

The answer seems to lie in how each chose to approach the data. According to statisticians at the Mayo Clinic, who compared the two analyses, "a reclassification of subjects by age" (Dr. Wolfe's analysis included all 50-year-olds with breast cancer in the younger group, making it appear that more DES mothers developed cancer at a younger age, whereas the Chicago analysis included these women in the older group) and "a redefinition of cases to be included account for most of the difference between the results of the two analyses (Wolfe vs. Chicago doctors)."

The Mayo statisticians explained further that the Wolfe analysis excluded several cases of breast cancer in control group mothers because the original pathology specimens were not available for review and double-checking. This meant *fewer* cases of breast cancer among control group mothers appeared in the Wolfe analysis, accentuating the difference between the control group and the DES-exposed group of mothers.

In addition, in analyzing the overall cancer incidence, the Wolfe analysis *included* 10 cases of cervical cancer (three in the control group and seven in the DES group) that the Chicago doctors *excluded* from their analysis, again adding weight to Wolfe's conclusion that DES increased a woman's risk for developing these cancers. Dr. Marion Hubby, DES project coordinator at the University of Chicago, emphasized, however, that the 10 cases were excluded from analysis because those cervical cancers were *not* the hormone-dependent type. I sought to clarify Dr. Wolfe's different approach, but he was "unavailable" when I contacted his office.

Dr. Wolfe generally defended his method of analyzing the Chicago data in a statement to the Food and Drug Administration that followed shortly after his letter to Secretary Califano. Wolfe stated: "In response to a request to Dr. Adrian Gross of the Food and Drug Administration's Bureau of Drugs to examine my evaluation of the data, he wrote me . . . that 'I find the statistical statements made in your letter to Secretary Califano to be quite appropriate. If it is true, as you tell me, that the University of Chicago people maintain these data do not demonstrate any kind of association between DES and cancer in women exposed to it in this particular study, I would judge such statements to be nothing short of absolute nonsense.' "

Sidney Wolfe also told the FDA that, based on his analysis of the Chicago data, there would be roughly 13,000 to 40,000 *more* cases of breast cancer among the estimated two million women who were given DES, depending upon the actual total dosage of DES given.

Lending credence to the Bibbo-Herbst conclusions is the fact that their paper with its conclusions was published in the *New England Journal of Medicine,* among the most respected medical journals in the world. Although nothing is infallible, it is true that all papers considered for publication in the *NEJM* are submitted to a rigorous review process *before* a decision is made to publish. It is highly unlikely that the journal editors would fail to notice incorrect data analysis, especially in a paper as important as this one. Finally, it is helpful to remember that a statistician can extract many findings—some conflicting—from a single set of data, depending on how the data are approached; that is, the classifications into which the data are broken. This is essentially what happened with the Chicago DES mothers data.

Drawn, in part, by the controversy over the possible significance of the Chicago data, six staff members of the Mayo Clinic (where, in the forties and fifties, a large number of pregnant women had been given DES) decided to do a retrospective breast cancer study of another set of DES mothers. Five of the six are members of the Mayo Clinic's Department of Medical Statistics and Epidemiology and the sixth is a professor of the clinic's Department of Obstetrics and Gynecology. These six investigators traced 408 women who had been given DES at the Mayo Clinic during their pregnancies. Eight of these women had confirmed cases of breast cancer compared to an expected number of slightly more than eight cases. The expected number of cases was extrapolated from mothers not exposed to DES in the local population. In other words, the Mayo Clinic DES mothers did not develop breast cancer any more frequently than their nonexposed counterparts.

The paper reporting the Mayo Clinic's breast cancer study was succinctly titled, "Breast Cancer in DES-Exposed Mothers: Absence of Association," and was published in the February 1980 issue of the *Mayo Clinic Proceedings*. The paper did essentially two things—it brought up the possibility that an increased risk for DES-related breast cancer might be dose-related (the more DES a woman took, presumably the greater her risk), and it elucidated the disagreement between Sidney Wolfe and the University of Chicago group, underscoring the uncertainty that still existed about DES mothers and breast cancer.

Of a dose-related increase in risk of breast cancer for DES mothers, the authors pointed out that the average total dose of DES given to women at the Mayo Clinic was considerably lower than that given at the University of Chicago—1.5 grams at the Mayo Clinic versus 11 to 12 grams at the University of Chicago. This, the Mayo Clinic doctors conjectured, may have been the reason that there were no more cases of breast cancer among their DES mothers than in the unexposed population. But as of this writing, no additional studies have been published that either prove or disprove this theory.

So, if neither the Wolfe analysis nor the Chicago analysis was incorrect, who is right? Despite the fact that it is obviously possible to extract opposite conclusions from the same set of data, what cannot be argued are the percentages of women in each group who got cancer.

It *is* a fact that 32 of 693 (4.6 percent) DES-treated mothers in the Chicago study developed breast cancer, compared to 21 of 668 (3.1 percent) women from the control group. It *is* a fact that four DES mothers developed ovarian cancer compared to only one woman in the control group. It *is* a fact that seven DES mothers compared to three in the control group developed cervical cancer. It *is* a fact that overall, 9.5 percent of the

DES mothers developed some form of cancer as compared to 6.9 percent of the control group mothers. It *is* a fact that the DES mothers with breast cancer developed the disease on an average of five years earlier than the control-group mothers with the disease. And, finally, it *is* a fact that more DES mothers with breast cancer died of their disease than did control group mothers.

Although the statistical significance of these data may continue to be disputed, the numbers themselves are unarguable. DES mothers in the University of Chicago study did have more breast, ovarian, colon, and cervical cancers than their counterparts in the control group.

One other, somewhat different, and much smaller study has been done that is also suggestive of an increased risk of cancer—specifically, of the ovaries—in women who took DES. Dr. Robert Hoover, head of Environmental Studies of the Division of Cancer Cause and Prevention of the National Cancer Institute, published a paper in a 1977 issue of *Lancet* (a highly respected English medical journal) reporting a larger than expected incidence of ovarian cancer in post-menopausal women treated with DES as estrogen replacement therapy. Dr. Hoover further reported an even greater risk of developing ovarian cancer if the women had taken DES and Premarin (a frequently prescribed brand of estrogens) simultaneously. This study, however, cannot be considered statistically significant (the number of cancers *could* be due to chance alone) since the numbers of women studied here were relatively small. In other words, there was not enough evidence to prove conclusively that the hormones the women had taken were responsible for their ovarian cancers. However, Dr. Hoover and his coauthors concluded that the results were highly "suggestive" and deserved further study.

While the women in the Hoover study were menopausal—a time in life when there is a striking natural alteration in the body's hormones and a time when the natural incidence of cancer increases—it should be remembered that these women received much smaller doses of DES than those given to pregnant women. The results of this study are yet another reminder of the powerful carcinogenic potential of DES.

Practically speaking, what do these conflicting opinions and confusing statistical analyses mean for DES mothers? Are they or are they not at increased risk for developing cancer, especially of the breast, and—more important—what can they do to help themselves?

## • DES MOTHERS AND BREAST CANCER

First, from the information we have so far, it appears that DES mothers *may* have a somewhat higher than average chance of developing breast cancer. It should be remembered that, *on the average,* one out of every 11 American women will develop breast cancer, according to the American Cancer Society, making it the most frequently occurring kind of cancer in American women and the leading cause of death from cancer in women. According to Barbara Seaman, coauthor of *Women and the Crisis in Sex Hormones,* that average risk is doubled if a woman has taken birth control pills for at least one year, or, roughly, an increase in risk to one out of six chances.

In a much publicized press release, Sidney Wolfe projected that DES mothers had a 75 percent higher than average risk of developing breast cancer. Many DES mothers who heard this figure panicked. Seventy-five percent is a walloping big number and for those women not good at math, that "75 percent" gave the impression that most DES mothers were bound to get breast cancer. This is simply not true. Translated, a 75 percent higher risk means a risk that is less than double or 1 chance in 7 to 8 compared with the average 1 in 11. This is less than the one Barbara Seaman projects for Pill users.

However, Dr. Wolfe has reportedly revised this risk estimate downward to less than a 40 percent higher risk; that is, a 1 out of 9 chance for DES mothers developing breast cancer.

Although DES was first implicated in the development of breast cancer as long ago as 1938 (*see* chapter 2, page 26, Lacassagne report)—the same year that DES was discovered—little information has come to light about how DES alters normal breast tissue. We know, for example, that certain conditions such as fibrocystic disease or a family history of breast cancer predispose a woman to the disease. It is also known that women whose bodies produce lower than average levels of progesterone (so that their estrogen-progesterone ratio is unnaturally weighted in favor of the estrogen in their bodies) are also at higher than average risk for breast cancer. According to Dr. David Rose, a specialist in the relationship between hormones and cancer, these women would also tend to have more problem pregnancies than average as well as more breast cancer.

Recently, a University of Wisconsin expert diagnostician of breast diseases, Dr. Raul Matallana, made another observation that may eventually help to explain how estrogens, and DES in particular, may cause precancerous and cancerous changes in breast tissue. During a review of follow-up mammograms (x-rays of the breast) taken of women who had already undergone one mastectomy and who had been placed on DES therapy (paradoxically, DES is successful in reducing the growth of some advanced breast cancers), Dr. Matallana noted that the tissue in the remaining breasts looked much denser than it had on mammograms taken *before* DES treatment was started. Since denser breast tissue, especially in older women, is associated with a higher incidence of breast cancer, Dr. Matallana was alarmed by what he saw. Although he stressed that this is a preliminary observation and is, as yet, unpublished, it is startling enough to warrant further investigation. Dr. Matallana would like to find out if this apparently DES-induced density is reversible upon cessation of DES therapy or if it is a permanent condition.

What is especially frightening about this observation is that the dose of DES that cancer patients receive is minuscule compared to the average daily as well as overall doses of DES received by DES mothers. Breast cancer patients take about 5 milligrams of DES daily over a period of perhaps several months, depending on their individual conditions. The dose of DES recommended by Drs. George and Olive Smith to prevent miscarriage (and the dose that hundreds of thousands of women received) started at 5 milligrams daily and was gradually increased throughout pregnancy to 175 milligrams daily. The total, overall dose many pregnant women received averaged a whopping 11,000 to 12,000 milligrams!

If breast tissue density increases with doses as small as 5 milligrams daily, what might happen to breast tissue under the influence of 10, 20, or 30 times that daily dose?

Even from these bits and pieces of information, it seems abundantly clear that DES mothers should avoid any further exposure to estrogen treatments. As Joseph Califano stated in his DES Advisory, no one knows if the effects of hormones are cumulative (*see* chapter 4). This includes estrogen replacement therapy to alleviate the symptoms of menopause, the "morning-after" birth control pill, DES to suppress lactation following the birth of a baby, or estrogenic birth control pills. (There is some evidence, however, that the newer birth control pills, which are predominantly made of progesterone-like compounds, may actually reduce a woman's risk for developing breast and uterine cancers.)

The deleterious effects of DES may well be cumulative and may set the stage for malignancies decades after exposure. It is important to note that estrogenic compounds other than DES also pose a potential increased hazard and should be avoided as well. This risk has been demonstrated in numerous animal studies as well as in humans where the increased incidence of cervical and endometrial cancers has been observed in post-menopausal women receiving estrogen replacement therapy. Although estrogen replacement therapy does temporarily relieve hot flashes and vaginal dryness, it is not a cure for menopause. Nor is menopause a disease that needs curing!

## Monthly Breast Self-Examinations

The American Cancer Society estimates that 111,000 American women will develop breast cancer in 1981 and roughly one-third of them will eventually die of their disease. Because early detection is the best chance a woman has for a cure, monthly breast self-examination is among the most important good health habits a woman can develop. Still, every woman who performs self-examination approaches it with a certain amount of dread. The fear is ever present that if one goes looking for a lump, one will eventually find one. Sylvia is the middle-aged mother of three daughters. Despite her keen intelligence and quick wit, she frankly admits that self-examination scares her. "I kind of dab a bit at each breast, then say, 'Thank God' to myself when I don't find anything."

But, as they say in the advertisements, it's the lumps you *don't* find that should scare you. So, first understand that your discomfiture at performing monthly self-examination is natural and normal. Second, note that 80 percent of breast lumps are benign. But, you should consult your doctor about all lumps and irregularities.

The best time to perform monthly self-examination is from four to seven days after the onset of your period, when the breasts are least likely to be tender. If you have passed your menopause, then choose the same time each month. The following description of breast self-examination is reprinted from publication No. 80-649 of the National Institutes of Health, published in August 1980 and titled "Breast Self-Examination."

A. LOOKING. Stand in front of a mirror with the upper body unclothed. Look for changes in the shape and size of the breasts and for dimpling of the skin or "pulling in" of the nipples. Any changes in the breast may be made more noticeable by a change in the position of the body and arms. So, look for any of the above signs or for changes in shape from one breast to another.

1. Stand with arms down.

2. Lean forward.

3. Raise arms overhead and press hands behind your head.

4. Place hands on hips and tighten chest and arm muscles by pressing firmly inward.

B. FEELING. Lie flat on your back with a pillow or folded towel under your shoulders and feel each breast with the opposite hand in sequence. With the hand slightly cupped, feel with flattened finger tips for lumps or any change in the texture of the breast or skin; also, note any discharge from nipples or scaling of the skin of the nipples. Feel gently, firmly, carefully, and thoroughly. Do not pinch your breast between thumb and fingers. This may give the impression of a lump that is not actually there.

1. Place a pillow or folded towel under your left shoulder. This raises the breast and makes examination easier. Place your left arm over your head. With your right hand, feel the inner half of your left breast from top to bottom and from nipple to breastbone.

2. Feel the outer half from bottom to top and from the nipple to the side of the chest.

3. Pay special attention to the area between the breast and armpit itself.

4. Now, place the pillow or folded towel under your right shoulder. Repeat this same process for your right breast using the fingers of your left hand to feel.

If you find something that you consider abnormal, contact your doctor for an examination. Dimpling or puckering of the skin of the breast or aureola (the dark skin around the nipple), a fluid discharge from the nipples, or a lump are all sufficient reasons to seek medical attention.

The chances are your doctor will recommend one or more of the following additional examinations to determine the nature of the lump or irregularity.

*Mammogram.* Mammography is an x-ray procedure of the

breast that has been widely used as both a general screening procedure and as a diagnostic tool when a breast lump or other irregularity has been found. A great deal of controversy has surrounded the use of mammography as a screening tool, primarily because it exposes thousands of women with no symptoms of breast disease to x-rays which, by themselves, some studies have indicated, might increase the chances for developing breast cancer.

However, in recent years improved radiographic equipment has made possible a much lower radiation dose per mammographic examination than was previously possible. With today's equipment, a woman need not be exposed to more than 1 rad (*r*adiation *a*bsorbed *d*ose) per breast per examination. According to Dr. George Fuller of Georgetown University Hospital, at this rate it would take 20 breast examinations to significantly increase a woman's risk for developing breast cancer.

Add to this the fact that mammography is a highly accurate diagnostic tool, and the value of the technique can readily be appreciated. According to a special report issued by the NIH-NCI (National Institutes of Health, National Cancer Institute), 95 percent of 592 minimal (very small) breast cancers were detected by mammography in 445,048 women studied.

Still, there are specific guidelines that should help a woman make a decision about whether or not to undergo routine mammography. The American Cancer Society published their recommendations concerning breast examination in July 1980. The society recommends that:

—All women over the age of 20 years perform monthly breast self-examination. In addition, women between the ages of 20 and 40 years should have a breast physical examination performed by a physician every three years, and women over 40 should have a breast physical examination annually.

—All women have a baseline mammogram by the age of 40. This can be extremely helpful as a comparison in evaluating subsequent changes in breast tissue should an irregularity develop.

—Women over 50 years have a mammogram every year; the radiation should be low-dose, below 1 rad for two views and preferably, below one-half a rad. [Women should not hesitate to ask about the number of rads they will be exposed to *prior* to mammography. Keep in mind that all x-ray equipment is not optimal; if the dose of radiation you will be exposed to exceeds optimal limits, seek another radiologist or another medical center.]

—Women between 40 and 50 years of age who have a personal or family history of breast cancer should have routine mammograms and should consult their physicians about the frequency of such examinations.

—Women below the age of 40 should have mammographic examinations only if there is a personal history of breast cancer. [This is because the risks associated with radiation may be higher in younger women, first because they have more years left to live, allowing more time for radiation-induced cancer to develop, and second, because their breast tissue is more dense than that of older women, providing less contrast between normal and abnormal tissue and making the mammogram more difficult to interpret accurately.]

When performed by experts, mammography is a valuable diagnostic tool and is the *only* method of detecting just-beginning cancers that are still too small to feel. If you have a lump or other symptom, you should not refuse to have a diagnostic mammogram.

Dr. Matallana stresses that mammography should be done in combination with a thorough breast physical examination performed by the doctor who interprets the mammogram. He says that subtle differences between the way a breast lump looks on a mammogram and the way it feels can offer valuable clues about the nature of the lesion.

"For example," he says, "benign lesions have similar di-

mensions both clinically and radiographically, whereas malignant lesions tend to appear smaller on mammograms, but feel
larger."

*Ultrasound examination.* Another diagnostic technique that
can be valuable in detecting breast disease is ultrasonography.
The distinct advantage of this technique is that it does not
involve the use of radiation, but rather, relies on sound waves.
However, because ultrasound technology is relatively new,
both the necessary equipment for breast examinations and
physicians with expertise in its use are still not widely available outside major medical centers.

Dr. Matallana stresses that ultrasound examination done by
a breast disease expert in concert with mammography and
physical examination has a diagnostic accuracy rate approach-
ing 100 percent, higher than for any single method alone.

The value of such a multiple approach is that in the case of
a benign breast lump, it can save the woman from having to
undergo the discomfort and trauma of biopsy surgery.

## What If It Looks Like Cancer?

If your physical examination, mammography, and ultrasound
examination (if you have had one) still leave room for doubt
or if they indicate a malignancy, your doctor will order a
biopsy, a surgical procedure in which the lump or suspicious
area of tissue is cut out. This is frequently performed with the
woman under full, or general, anesthesia, but depending on
the location of the lump, can be done with local anesthesia.

If you are scheduled to undergo a biopsy under general
anesthesia, *remember you have options.*

First, consider the surgery itself. Most often, doctors will
perform "one-step" surgery; this means that your breast lump
will be removed and, while you are still under anesthesia and
on the operating table, the lump will be frozen and sent to a
waiting pathologist for immediate analysis. This examination
takes roughly 15 minutes. If the lump proves malignant, your

surgeon will then proceed immediately to perform a mastectomy.

This one-step surgery is favored by physicians because the patient avoids a second surgical procedure and a second exposure to anesthesia. (About one in one thousand patients will die as a result of a general anesthetic, no matter how simple the surgical procedure.)

However, it is important to remember the emotional trauma associated with the "one-step" mastectomy—being "put to sleep" for a diagnostic procedure (the biopsy) and knowing you might wake up with half your chest cut away. The one-step surgery leaves no opportunity for patient and doctor to discuss the nature or extent of the malignancy or the options for treatment.

In her book *No More Menstrual Cramps and Other Good News,* Dr. Penny Wise Budoff makes a strong argument for a "two-step" surgical procedure. She recommends that if the biopsy indicates that the lump is malignant, the patient should have the mastectomy at a later date and in a separate surgical procedure. She writes, "I have always felt that this combined procedure, while it is very convenient for the surgeon, leaves room for irreversible error and needlessly subjects patients—most of whom will prove not to have cancer—to anxiety and fear."

With a two-step procedure, the pathologist then has time to examine a tissue specimen more extensively, noting the type of cancer, and whether it's slow or fast-growing, localized or invasive. Then the woman can decide with her doctor what form of surgery and post-operative treatment will be best for her.

Two types of mastectomy are most frequently performed in the United States. The radical, or Halsted, procedure (named after the surgeon who devised it) involves removing the cancerous breast, lymph glands (nodes) under the arm, and the underlying chest muscle. The modified radical mastectomy means removing the breast and some of the lymph glands, leaving the underlying muscle intact. The Halsted procedure, introduced near the turn of the century and the method of choice for the last 80 years, is now losing its popularity in the medical community. Whereas doctors had believed this radical surgery offered a woman the best chance of a cure for her breast cancer, studies in recent years have shown *no difference in survival* between women who have had the radical as compared to the modified radical mastectomy.

If your doctor tells you he plans to perform a radical mastectomy, *go to another doctor!* The radical surgery not only grossly disfigures a woman's chest, but leaves her arm swollen and weak from extensive loss of lymph glands and muscle. Because a modified radical mastectomy causes significantly less disfigurement and debilitation, with no demonstrable loss of her chances for a cure, a woman is well advised to consider this less extensive surgery.

Most recently, doctors have been studying the results of performing a simple mastectomy (removal of the breast only), followed by radiation therapy to kill any lingering microscopic traces of cancer. The results of this approach have been extremely promising with women who have early-stage cancers, and should be considered another treatment possibility.

Simple lumpectomy—removal of the tumor alone, leaving the breast—followed by radiation is yet a fourth option. Although this procedure is by far the most cosmetically acceptable, it has yet to be proven that it will work as well as the more extensive surgeries to eradicate breast cancer. However, there are a number of surgeons who are now advocating this approach for patients with small tumors.

Surgery, radiation, and chemotherapy, including hormones, are all part of medical science's arsenal in fighting breast cancer. The important thing for you to remember if you develop breast cancer is that *you have a choice about how you are to be treated.* Take the time to exercise your options. You will have to live with the results for the rest of your life. Don't be afraid to question your doctor and surgeon about all treatment possibilities. If you are not satisfied with the answers you get, by all means visit another doctor for a second opinion.

## Breast Reconstruction

For a woman who has undergone a mastectomy, her missing breast can be a continual reminder of illness and pain. Breast reconstruction, although not "perfect," *can* restore normal body contours and so help her to regain her sense of well-being.

I offer the following information (for which I am indebted to Dr. Richard Dowden, a plastic surgeon and breast reconstruction specialist at the Cleveland Clinic) as an introduction to this restorative procedure.

*What is breast reconstruction?* Breast reconstruction is the surgical recreation of a breast using a silicone implant and the patient's own skin and muscle. Reconstruction may be done in one operation or may require several operative steps, depending on the extent of a woman's mastectomy (radical, modified radical, or simple). If a great deal of tissue was removed to begin with, then muscle-skin grafts may be necessary as a separate operation before a silicone implant can be placed.

*Who should have a breast reconstruction?* Nearly every woman who has undergone a mastectomy can also undergo breast reconstruction. Breast reconstruction will *not* cause a cancer to return, although there are a small number of women who— for various medical reasons—may be advised *not* to have this surgery.

*What is a reconstructed breast like?* "A reconstructed breast," stresses Dr. Dowden, "is not a normal breast." It is usually firmer and flatter against the chest wall, is scarred from surgery, and is often not accepted by a woman's partner as a normal sexual feature. It also lacks the sensitivity to touch of a normal breast.

However, while the reconstructed breast will not look normal when a woman is unclothed, it *will* look and feel normal when the woman is dressed. "And," adds Dr. Dowden, "because the reconstruction is such a big improvement over the mastectomy deformity, women are usually quite pleased with the results."

*When can breast reconstruction be done?* Only in recent years have newer surgical techniques made breast reconstruction feasible for most women. As a result, many women who had mastectomies years ago may think that it is too late for them. This is definitely not so. Breast reconstruction can be performed at any time after the mastectomy—days, months, and even years later.

*Insurance repayments for breast reconstruction.* Although many insurance companies now cover the cost of breast reconstruction following mastectomy for cancer, some companies still consider this surgery "cosmetic." Dr. Dowden, whose paper on insurance repayments for breast reconstruction appeared in *JAMA* (*Journal of the American Medical Association*) in 1979, believes strongly that sexual discrimination underlies much of the refusal to reimburse a woman for the cost of reconstruction. He says that cosmetic surgery is defined as "operating to change some feature of the body that is already in the normal range. No one," he stresses, "could honestly consider the mastectomy deformity to be within the range of normal." Also, Dr. Dowden says, many of the same companies that have refused repayment for breast reconstruction have allowed repayment for a testicular implant following the loss of a testicle through disease or injury.

Women who have been denied even partial repayment for breast reconstruction should contact their state insurance commissioners for assistance. Surgeons, Dr. Dowden says, can also help by contacting senior insurance company executives when a claim is denied because "many misunderstandings may occur at the lower levels of corporate bureaucracy."

Not every woman undergoing a mastectomy will choose

breast reconstruction, but every woman should know that this restorative surgery is an entirely reasonable option available to her. Perhaps just knowing that she need not go through life with a major deformity in case of mastectomy will make a woman less reluctant to seek early, life-saving medical attention for breast cancer symptoms.

For more detailed information about breast diseases and treatments, get a copy of the booklet "If You've Thought About Breast Cancer," by Rose Kushner (full address in appendix). It gives clear, concise information written by a professional medical writer who also happens to be a DES mother and a former breast cancer patient. Dr. Budoff's book, *No More Menstrual Cramps,* etc., published by G. P. Putnam's Sons, also contains an excellent discussion of breast diseases and treatment options.

## Relieving Benign Cystic Breast Disease

Because DES mothers may well be at a slightly increased risk for developing breast cancer as are women with benign fibrocystic disease (noncancerous lumps in the breast), they should take whatever steps they can to reduce that risk. The following measures were found to reduce or eliminate fibrocystic disease, and perhaps the attendant increased risk for breast cancer (although they have not yet been *shown* to reduce the risk for breast cancer).

The first treatment involves the elimination from a woman's diet those foods and beverages that contain chemicals known as methylxanthines. These foods include tea, coffee, cola, chocolate, and some decongestant remedies. Even decaffeinated coffee and herbal teas have some methylxanthines (caffeine, theophylline, and theobromine). This group of chemicals interferes with a natural enzyme process, resulting in increased breast cell growth and the formation of breast cysts and fibrous tissue. Marilyn, a DES mother with longstanding fibrocystic disease, tried the diet for six months. "It works!" she exclaimed, but eventually she drifted back to her morning cups of coffee, and experienced a return of her breast lumps.

Dr. John Peter Minton of the Department of Surgery at Ohio State University College of Medicine has pioneered this method of treating breast cysts. In a recent study, he reported that 37 out of 45 women who stopped all methylxanthine consumption had complete resolution of their breast disease. Only one woman in this group showed no improvement! The rest had partial improvement. In another group of women who reduced, but did not eliminate, the offending foods from their diets, fibrocystic disease disappeared in one-quarter of the women, was reduced in another one-half, and was not affected in the remaining one-quarter. Dr. Minton also found that smokers were less likely to benefit from the methylxanthine-free diet.

The second treatment consists of taking 600 international units daily of vitamin E. Dr. Robert S. London, assistant professor of obstetrics and gynecology at Johns Hopkins University School of Medicine, found that more than one-third of the women who took vitamin E daily for four weeks found their breast lumps had disappeared. Another 40 percent had partial resolution of their cystic disease—improvement but not elimination. The remaining women experienced no change. It should be added, however, that vitamin E also appears to affect fatty metabolism, and may have other, as yet unknown, effects on the body. Because of these unknowns, the vitamin E treatment must still be labeled "experimental."

*Other Physical Conditions Associated with DES Mothers*

Besides a possible increased risk of developing breast cancer, DES mothers may suffer from other diseases, not all malignant, but still causing distress and disability.

For years, DES Action chapters all over the country have heard stories from many DES mothers about their endocrine disorders. Trouble is, no formal medical inquiry was ever made into a possible association between DES ingestion in humans and endocrine problems. Coupled with the often hard-to-pinpoint symptoms of endocrine unbalance, it has been all too easy for some physicians to categorize women with such complaints as "crocks" and "neurotics." Other women report drifting from one doctor to another in an often fruitless search for someone who can help them. And, all too often, yet others were given birth control pills or subjected to hysterectomies or both as a simplistic cure-all for "those female complaints."

However, animal studies have shown that at least two endocrine glands can malfunction in the presence of DES. For example, three Pennsylvania State University researchers recently found that lambs implanted with DES suffered a marked diminution of thyroid activity as well as a thickening (hyperplasia) of the adrenal cortex. Both these effects result in significant ill health. (*See* chapter 2 for detailed discussions of the thyroid and adrenal glands, and chapter 1 for an account of my own experience with hypothyroidism.)

While I caution the reader against self-diagnosis, this information may help some women to help themselves by knowing the possible effects of their DES exposure.

For additional health care guidelines for DES mothers, see chapter 7 and the DES Task Force recommendations.


## • DEALING WITH THE EMOTIONAL IMPACT OF BEING A DES MOTHER

Being a DES mother—to paraphrase a popular platitude—means always saying you're sorry. *Fear* ("My child might get cancer!"), *guilt* ("I did this to my child!"), and indelible *regret* ("How I wish I'd never taken it!") stain the peace of mind of most DES mothers, and sometimes leave a lasting blotch of mistrust on the delicate fabric of the mother-daughter relationship.

To cope effectively with this triple-headed emotional hydra, DES mothers must face their feelings honestly. Unlike the nine-headed Hydra of Greek mythology, which grew back two heads for every one cut off, the three-headed DES hydra grows more fearsome only if it is ignored. Unfortunately, it is all too human to want to ignore any kind of unhappy situation. The psychiatrists call it "denial." When I miscarried, for example, in those fleeting moments immediately following the loss of the fetus, I soothed myself with the lie that what came out of me was just some superfluous tissue and that a baby was still growing inside of me. For those few moments, I could not bring myself to face the profound sense of loss I inevitably felt, so I denied the loss completely.

For a distinct number of DES mothers, denial of the DES threat *is* the way they cope with their personal "hydras." But, these mothers are only kidding themselves, and what is worse, they are putting the health of their children in further jeopardy.

Many other mothers will acknowledge the dangers of DES exposure to themselves, but will withhold knowledge of DES exposure from their affected children. One mother wrote, "My daughter is a student in advanced graduate studies. I would prefer not to involve her in examinations or discussions about DES if, in view of her age, the danger period is past." This mother and others like her risk not only their daughters' health (since these women should be checked for the rest of their lives), but flirt with the danger of doing irreparable harm to their relationships with their children. DES mothers should ask themselves how their daughters would react if they knew their mothers were keeping vital health information from them.

DES mothers of sons seem somewhat more reluctant to discuss their exposure than women of daughters, perhaps because less has been written about sons or because no cancers have been directly associated with DES in sons, or perhaps because, in spite of our society's great push for sexual equality, it is still far less acceptable to discuss male genital problems than to talk about female problems.

Whatever the reasons, the advice for mothers of sons is the same as for those women who have daughters. First, be honest with yourself and with your children. In one of only two papers published to date on the psychological effects of DES exposure, Dr. Ruth Schwartz of the University of Rochester wrote that DES daughters who coped best with the anxiety attendant to their DES exposure were usually those whose mothers had first told them about DES. Generally, these mother and daughters also had close relationships and good lines of communication.

Second, DES mothers should be realistic. Remember, that in spite of the fact that the vast majority of DES daughters have benign abnormalities of the reproductive organs, only a fraction will develop adenocarcinoma. Many more may have problems having babies of their own, but in time, these problems, too, may yield to increased medical knowledge and awareness of the problems. And, bear in mind, too, that according to recent studies, the large majority of DES daughters who want to will eventually bear a child in spite of previous miscarriages. One 27-year-old DES daughter had six miscarriages but finally gave birth to a healthy, eight-pound baby boy.

Third, talk with other DES mothers and their children. It will help you to know you are not alone and that your fears and feelings of guilt can be surmounted.

# 7 · The Government Response to DES— A Chronology

*"Those concerned about drug risks and over-use want the FDA to be cautious in approving new drugs. Those who emphasize the medical benefits of drug therapy often accuse the FDA of excessive caution. . . . Actually, there can be truth in both positions."*

DONALD KENNEDY, *Ph.D., president of Stanford University and former Commissioner of the Food and Drug Administration (1977–1979)*

The Food and Drug Administration (FDA), which is charged with protecting us from unsafe and ineffective food-stuffs and drugs is—like many government agencies—a leviathan. With well over 7,000 employees laboring to investigate, enforce, define, clarify, test, and approve or disapprove thousands of items yearly, the FDA can be a ponderously slow beast. And slow it was to restrict the use of DES.

In 1940, when the FDA approved DES for use in humans, few criteria existed for judging new drugs. The 1906 Pure Food and Drug Act gave enforcement as well as advisory capabilities to the fledgling bureau that eventually became the FDA. It also gave consumers some assurance that the medications and foodstuffs they bought were correctly labeled, and that those contents were not grossly adulterated. In 1938, more detailed federal guidelines were drawn up to help assure that foods, drugs, and cosmetics were safe for human consumption.

However, the medical sciences in general were still young, and an awareness that drugs could pose long-term dangers was virtually nonexistent. So, the 1938 guidelines did not include the need for drug companies to demonstrate long-range safety; nor did they require proof of effectiveness. It was not until 1962 that new Congressional drug regulation laws required manufacturers to prove effectiveness as well as safety. For DES, this meant a belated re-evaluation.

For nearly three decades following its initial approval of DES, the FDA never questioned the drug—not even after the University of Chicago study, which was published in 1953, showed that DES was useless in preventing miscarriage despite the fact that millions of prescriptions of DES were being written for this purpose.

When drug regulations were tightened in 1962, the FDA sought to review the thousands of drugs it had approved prior to that time. Enlisting the help of the National Academy of Sciences to evaluate these older drugs, the FDA asked that the drugs be judged either "probably effective" or "possibly effective." Bear in mind that they had already been judged "safe." For those drugs found "possibly effective," the onus of proving effectiveness was to be placed on the drug manufacturer. If no such proof was forthcoming within six months, the FDA was empowered to restrict the use of that drug.

In 1967 the National Academy of Sciences wrote that DES was "possibly effective" as an antiabortive agent. Although the burden of proof was then shifted to the drug companies, six months came, then went, and the manufacturers of DES still submitted no proof of its effectiveness in preventing miscarriage. In spite of this, for reasons that are not clear, the FDA did not restrict the use of DES during pregnancy despite its own rule about the six-month grace period. (Had it done so, I would not have been given DES in 1969.) There is additional evidence that the FDA was slow to act even after Dr. Herbst and his colleagues gave proof early in 1971 to then commissioner of the FDA, Dr. Charles Edwards, that DES given during pregnancy could cause cancer in the female offspring.

In their book *Women and the Crisis in Sex Hormones,* Barbara and Gideon Seaman state that "the FDA took no steps to restrict DES use in pregnancy until November 1971." This was a full seven months after receiving the Herbst Report which irrefutably connected DES given during pregnancy with vaginal cancer in seven DES daughters. Then, the FDA finally issued a ruling requiring the drug companies to warn against the use of DES during pregnancy. This was four years after the FDA asked the National Science Foundation to determine DES's effectiveness in preventing miscarriage and 18 years after the Dieckmann study showed DES to be ineffective as an antiabortive agent.

By the time the government was to make its next major move regarding DES, the cancer scare had grown considerably.

### • 1973: THE DESAD PROJECT

In December 1973, another government agency, the National Cancer Institute, a branch of the Department of Health, Education, and Welfare (now known as the Department of Health and Human Services), started the ball rolling toward a formal study of DES use during pregnancy. The resulting study was dubbed the DESAD Project—short for DES adenosis. The basic purpose of the study was and remains "to assess the magnitude and severity of the health hazard to DES-exposed female offspring."

The DESAD Project was first proposed by Dr. Leonard Kurland, chairman of the Department of Epidemiology and Medical Statistics at the Mayo Clinic and now national coordinator of the DESAD project. Dr. Kurland reported in an interview that the idea for the project came after the Herbst-Ulfelder-Poskanzer article first reporting the DES-cancer connection. Alarmed because many Mayo Clinic patients had been given DES during pregnancy, Dr. Kurland and his staff rushed to review their own DES-exposed population. Because of their computerized information retrieval system, they quickly identified nearly 1,800 DES daughters born to women treated with DES at the Mayo Clinic.

Then began a systematic evaluation of these records, and based on the large size of the exposed population and the potential seriousness of the medical consequences (at that time, no one was sure how many DES daughters would develop cancer), they wrote a letter to the FDA for funding to conduct a preliminary study. The funding, they proposed, would help pay for the examinations of DES daughters and for the epidemiological evaluations. Dr. Kurland said that, much to his surprise and contrary to the stories he had heard of government unresponsiveness, within three weeks the FDA sent a check for $12,000 to the Mayo Clinic for the preliminary study outlined by Dr. Kurland.

Based on the results of this FDA-funded study, Dr. Kurland and his staff applied in 1973 to the National Cancer Institute for funds for a much larger, multi-institutional study. Dr. Kurland said that soon after doing the preliminary study, he realized that institutional differences in the timing and amounts of DES given to pregnant women, as well as more subtle environmental and ethnic differences in population, might result in different regional reactions to DES. For example, the Mayo Clinic generally prescribed much lower total doses of DES to pregnant women than did the University of Chicago or Boston physicians. (*See* chapter 6 for details of dosage differences as they relate to breast cancer in DES mothers.)

The result of the Mayo Clinic work and their petition to the National Cancer Institute (NCI) was the DESAD Project. In December 1973, the NCI announced plans to establish the multicenter project first proposed by Dr. Kurland and his staff to study DES daughters, and by March 1974, the contracts for this study were awarded.

The DESAD Project was set up as a "field test to answer questions concerning incidence, prevalence, and natural history" of changes in the vaginal tissues of DES daughters. This was to include a study of benign as well as malignant changes. Since it had already been established by 1974 that many DES daughters had benign abnormalities of the vaginal tissues (adenosis being the most prominent feature of these), it was important to find out if these abnormalities were precursors to cancer, as well as to determine what a DES daughter's actual risk was for developing vaginal cancer.

The National Cancer Institute chose four health care institutions as the DESAD Project's field participants, and the project was funded for three years for $3 million. The four institutions and their DESAD project directors are the Massachusetts General Hospital in Boston, Dr. Ann Barnes and Dr. Stanley Robboy; Baylor College of Medicine, Dr. Raymond H. Kaufman; University of Southern California, Dr. Duane Townsend; and the Mayo Clinic, Dr. David Decker. The Gunderson Clinic in La Crosse, Wisconsin, serves as an adjunct DESAD examination center for the Mayo Clinic. Dr. Kurland and his staff were appointed as the coordinating unit for the entire project.

Participating institutions were chosen for their proximity to a large, DES-exposed population, and for their ability in terms of equipment and professional staff to carry out the project's study plan. A minimum of 2,000 DES daughters with proven prenatal exposure to DES were enrolled in the project, half of whom were identified through a search of medical records. These patients found by record review are considered the most representative cross-section of DES daughters since they were chosen regardless of their medical conditions. The others were referred by physicians outside the study or were self-referred for participation in the DESAD project.

In addition to DES-exposed women, a minimum of 750 DES unexposed women were enrolled in the project to act as controls. Some of the controls are sisters of the DES daughters in the project. Others are young women chosen to match the DES-exposed women in terms of age, city of birth, and their mothers' prenatal problems. Most DESAD Project enrollees are now in their twenties with the eldest currently (1981) about 30 years of age.

The first collective findings of the DESAD Project were

submitted for publication in 1978 and published in early 1979. Briefly, they revealed that one-third of the daughters selected by record review had benign changes of the vaginal and cervical tissues as did two-thirds of the enrollees referred by physicians, and that the degree of these changes was associated with the week during pregnancy in which the mothers began taking DES. Second, it was found that these changes appeared to normalize as the DES daughters grew older, a now well-recognized phenomenon. Third, it was found that the risk for developing DES-related vaginal adenocarcinoma was lower than expected. (None of the record review enrollees has developed cancer.) The precise risk was calculated by Dr. Arthur Herbst, who is not an investigator in the DESAD Project, but who does maintain the national registry for DES-caused cancers (*see* chapter 3). During 1980, DESAD Project investigators also reported that DES daughters had a higher incidence of miscarriage than would normally be expected, although 80 percent of DES daughters who wanted a baby eventually bore a live child. (For more on this subject, *see* chapter 4.)

Although the National Cancer Institute renewed funding for the DESAD Project in 1977 for an additional five years, this contract is scheduled to expire in 1982. Project investigators are applying for additional five-year funding, but are concerned that government budget cutbacks might jeopardize the future of the project.

Dr. Kurland said during an interview that new problems, including a second peak incidence of invasive clear-cell cancer in DES daughters, might occur as the DES-exposed population grows older, and that such a trend could only be accurately assessed and appropriate treatments developed through a study such as the DESAD Project.

## *Other DES Studies Being Funded by the NCI*

In addition to the DESAD Project, the NCI is funding a three-year study at the Mayo Clinic to examine the effects of DES on the urogenital systems of exposed sons. Secondarily, fertility in the study population will be assessed. Dr. Lawrence Resseguie, the coordinator for this project, said that the findings, which involve 300 DES sons and an equal number of "controls," will be published early in 1982.

The NCI is also funding a multicenter project to assess the risk of breast cancer in DES mothers. The participating centers are Dartmouth-Hanover Medical Center, Baylor University College of Medicine, the Mayo Clinic, and the Massachusetts General Hospital. The principal investigator is Dr. Robert Greenberg of Dartmouth.

## • FEBRUARY TO SEPTEMBER 1978: THE DES TASK FORCE

Coincident with the publication of the DESAD Project's first findings was the formation of the DES Task Force, convened at the behest of Joseph Califano, then Secretary of the Department of Health, Education, and Welfare, and implemented by Dr. Julius Richmond, Surgeon-General of the United States. Composed of 14 physicians and researchers of the National Cancer Institute (an agency of HEW), the task force was charged with reviewing all aspects of the DES problem, and with making recommendations for health care of the exposed and research directions for medical investigators.

Califano also asked the task force members to specifically investigate the possibility of an increased risk of breast cancer in DES mothers, the use of DES as a "morning-after" birth control pill, abnormalities of the vaginal and cervical tissue in DES daughters, abnormalities of the urogenital tract in DES sons, and "other observations" on the health effects of DES.

Dr. Diane Fink, director of the Division of Cancer Control and Rehabilitation of the NCI, was appointed to head the task force. For six months, its members worked to sort out hundreds of bits of information and then to piece them together into one clear and telling whole. In addition to considering hundreds of scientific papers about various aspects of DES, the task force invited the testimony of physicians and others with expertise about DES.

In addition, task force members were guided by a panel of consultants, distinguished as much by the breadth and depth of their knowledge about DES as by their diverse perspectives. These consultants included Dr. Arthur Herbst, director of the DES cancer registry, senior author of the paper that first revealed the DES-cancer connection, and chairman of the Department of Obstetrics and Gynecology at the University of Chicago School of Medicine; Dr. Leonard Kurland, medical coordinator of the DESAD Project; and health-care consumer advocates Dr. Sidney Wolfe, and Barbara Seaman, author of *Women and the Crisis in Sex Hormones*. Two other consultants were DES mothers—Fran Fishbane, cofounder and former president of DES Action, and Phyllis Wetherill, who has spoken extensively about the effects of DES.

On September 21, 1978, six months after it began its investigation, the task force published its findings. These were divided into 10 sections beginning with an introduction and followed by discussions of DES daughters, DES mothers, DES sons, psychosocial implications of DES exposure, current uses of DES (and other estrogens), and recommendations for public and for professional education.

The following is a brief summary merely highlighting these findings.

• *SEPTEMBER 21, 1978: THE TASK FORCE FINDINGS*

For the sake of thorough documentation as well as the reader's convenience, I present the following synopsis of task force findings even though some of this information can be found elsewhere in this book.

The reader should bear in mind that the task force findings

and recommendations were collected and formulated in 1978. Although they remain remarkably accurate as far as they go, new information may come to light that may supersede that available to the task force.

*DES daughters.* The task force confirmed that a clear association exists between *in utero* exposure to DES and clear-cell adenocarcinoma of the vagina and cervix, and that the risk for any DES daughter developing this cancer is no greater than one chance in 700 nor less than one chance in 7,000. (*See* chapter 4 for more details.)

—Many DES daughters have benign, abnormal changes of the vagina and cervix. But there is nothing to indicate that these benign abnormalities are precancerous conditions.

—DES daughters do not seem to have an increased risk for developing *in situ* carcinomas as compared to unexposed women.

—There is some evidence to indicate that DES daughters may have infertility problems (*see* chapter 4 for a more current discussion of this subject), but no evidence to indicate that the babies of DES daughters have a higher rate of birth defects than the babies of unexposed women.

—Recommendations for health care of daughters include at least an annual pelvic examination and Pap smear (*see* chapter 4 for details), including a colposcopy at the first visit and at subsequent visits when the Pap smear is abnormal or if there are widespread tissue changes. Periodic screening should begin at age 14 or at the onset of menstruation, whichever comes first. Vaginal bleeding or discharge (other than menstruation) should be evaluated immediately, whenever it occurs. Biopsies should not be done routinely, but only when there is an abnormal Pap test or "significant epithelial abnormalities."

—Breast examinations should conform with current guidelines (*see* chapter 6).

For a complete discussion of medical guidelines for DES daughters, see chapter 4.

*DES mothers.* The task force expressed "serious concern

about the carcinogenic potential of DES in women who took the drug during pregnancy."

—It urged all DES mothers to inform their physicians of their DES exposure so that this fact can be taken into consideration in case of an abnormal finding. In general, the task force said that "*asymptomatic* DES mothers should be *urged* to follow a system of routine screening *which would be considered appropriate for women without prior estrogen exposure.*" This screening should include an annual pelvic examination and a Pap smear and a breast physical examination (*see* chapter 6 for complete guidelines).

—The task force mentioned that DES mothers and their physicians should be alerted that DES mothers may be at increased risk for developing breast cancer and that such cancer could develop at an earlier age than in unexposed women, or within 20 years of their exposure to DES.

—The task force also expressed concern about DES mothers undergoing mammography as a routine screening procedure because of a possibly synergistic effect between x-rays and DES in producing breast cancer. However, they recommended that mammography may be performed as a diagnostic procedure if there are signs and symptons suggestive of breast cancer.

*DES sons.* There is a suspicion that DES sons may have more abnormalities of the genital and lower urinary tract than other men. As of 1978, the task force found no definitive information on the fertility implications of abnormal urogenital findings in DES sons. (More on this subject in chapter 5.)

—DES sons should be informed of their exposure and should undergo a physical examination to check for abnormalities, such as undescended testicles, since these conditions occur more frequently in DES sons and since both these conditions are well-recognized as predisposing to testicular cancer.

—The task force found that evidence was inconclusive for a positive association with DES and infertility and DES and an increased risk of cancer. However, task force members felt that both these questions warranted further investigation. (See more recent information on male infertility in chapter 5.)

*Psychosocial implications.* The task force acknowledged that there might be substantial psychological and social stress resulting from DES exposure.

—It recommended that additional controlled studies be made of this problem in view of the paucity of information on the subject.

—It also urged physicians and other health professionals "to be aware and sensitive to the emotional impact of DES exposure" when examining or treating DES sons, mothers, or daughters, and suggested special counseling for those individuals experiencing substantial stress.

*Postcoital use (the "morning-after" pill).* The task force expressed serious reservations about DES as a "morning-after" birth control pill for reasons similar to those expressed in chapter 4.

—Further, task force members specified that DES-exposed women should avoid any further use of DES and other estrogens "when possible" since the cumulative effects of such exposures are unknown. They especially expressed concern over reports of frequent prescriptions for the "morning-after" pill for college students, and cautioned that such contraception should be "restricted to situations where no alternative is judged acceptable by a fully informed patient and her physician."

*Professional education.* The task force urged that its findings be sent to all physicians in the form of a summary report as a Physician Advisory from the Surgeon-General. In addition, it advised that these findings should be distributed for publication in widely circulated medical journals, such as the *Journal of the American Medical Association (JAMA)* and to professional society bulletins.

Specific task force recommendations included:

—A national list of physicians to be drawn up by professional societies from whom a second opinion might be obtained on DES problems.

—Special seminars at medical meetings on the health effects of DES.

—The development of educational materials about DES for nurses, social workers, and other health care professionals.

—Physician notification of all women for whom they prescribed DES during pregnancy and advice for follow-up care for both mothers and children, and a pointed suggestion that the physician provide this information free of charge.

*Public information.* Women who took DES during pregnancy and their sons and daughters should be informed of their exposure and the possible health consequences through notification by their physicians and through public information campaigns by appropriate agencies, such as state and local health departments.

*Reimbursement.* The task force recommended that the Secretary of Health, Education, and Welfare urge all health-insurance carriers to extend their coverage to include the cost of DES screening examinations, since it became apparent through testimony to the task force that many DES daughters had difficulty obtaining insurance coverage or reimbursement for periodic DES screening.

—The task force also urged careful consideration of government funding, among other sources, to pay the medical costs of individuals who are not covered by health insurance.

Although the task force and its findings emphatically express government concern over a monumental medical fiasco, many of the task force's recommendations—to wit, those requiring any sacrifice of time and/or money from physicians and insurance companies—have yet to be implemented.

For example, I have yet to meet a single DES mother whose DES-prescribing physician notified her of her exposure. Worse yet, many of these physicians refuse to cooperate when the women contact *them* for copies of their records. And, there are still (in 1981) numerous anecdotal reports of DES daughters unable to obtain insurance coverage or reimbursement for DES-related medical examinations. Nor have professional, medical societies yet drawn up a national list of physicians with DES expertise for referrals; *that* important job is being done painstakingly by the volunteers of DES Action, the national consumer group.

## October 4, 1978: Physician Advisory

Within two weeks of the task force release of its findings, Surgeon-General Julius Richmond issued a physician advisory summarizing the findings. The six-page advisory, which was sent to physicians all over the country, contained a recommendation that all physicians notify those patients to whom they had prescribed DES during pregnancy. As I mentioned above, few seem to have complied. Most women have learned of the DES problem through magazines, newspapers, and public service campaigns.

This advisory was remarkable because it was only the third cancer warning ever issued by the Surgeon-General, the first two involving cigarettes and asbestos.

## • DES AS A GROWTH STIMULANT FOR CATTLE

About the same time that DES became the rage as a treatment for threatened miscarriage, farmers started implanting their cattle and chickens with DES pellets to make them plumper, juicier, and more profitable at the market.

Although the FDA banned DES pellets implanted in the necks of chickens in 1959, when dangerously high levels of the drug were found in the consumable flesh of the birds, similar implants in cattle were allowed for 20 years more. On November 1, 1979, the FDA permanently banned the use of DES as a growth stimulant in cattle. This ban marked the legal end of a decade-long struggle between the Food and Drug Administration and the cattle breeders.

The idea of feeding (as opposed to implanting) DES to cattle was developed in 1954 at Iowa State University by Dr.

Wise Burroughs. In the July 1954 issue of *Science,* Dr. Burroughs wrote favorably about the effects of feeding DES to cattle. Despite this positive view of DES as a feed additive, Dr. Burroughs even then demonstrated an awareness and sensitivity to the possible adverse health effects on humans of consuming DES-laced meat. In advocating DES as a feed additive, Dr. Burroughs wrote that although the "advantages of diethylstilbestrol implantations have been known for some time," this method of administering DES could result in "a potential human health hazard ... if substantial pellet residues remain in the tissues of treated cattle at the time of slaughter." Dr. Burroughs continued that DES feed additives, by contrast, resulted in the "desirable effects of pellet implantation without any of the undesirable effects."

One year later, Dr. Burroughs obtained a patent on the use of DES feed additives for cattle on behalf of the Iowa State College Research Foundation. The income generated for the foundation by this patent has totaled $3,389,304.68, enough to fund a variety of research projects as well as the construction of an auditorium.

In spite of the widespread use of DES in cattle feed as indicated by the substantial revenues generated by the Iowa State patent, and despite Dr. Burrough's warnings about the potential health hazards of such implants, DES pellets eventually proved to be the more popular method of administering DES, and the use of this method continued unabated until 1979.

Although the FDA banned DES as a feed additive in August 1972 and as an implant in April 1973, feedlot owners managed to take successful legal action in the federal courts to block the implementation of these bans. However, as analytical methodology improved, substantial amounts of DES became detectable, which could not be found by older methods of analysis in the meat and especially in the liver and kidneys of DES-supplemented animals. Based on this new evidence, the FDA moved once again on November 1, 1979, and this time the ban stuck. But, so strong was the siren call of extra profits from super-fat, DES-boosted cattle that intransigent feedlot owners and cattle growers have, in a disturbing number of cases, stockpiled DES to feed and implant their cattle illegally.

During 1980, FDA inspectors found nearly half a million head of cattle illegally implanted with DES pellets and more than 1,200 cattle which had been illegally fed DES. The FDA has ordered the "reconditioning" of these cattle, which means that following the surgical removal of the pellets by a licensed veterinarian, cattle must be held for at least 35 days before slaughter to give the DES a chance to be excreted, and 63 days if the kidneys or liver are to be used.

Feedlot owners found guilty of illegally administering DES to their cattle risk FDA prosecution and up to a three-year term in prison and a $10,000 fine. To date, the FDA has found 115 feedlot owners who have illegally given their cattle DES.

Although DES may no longer be used legally for cattle or chickens, a number of other hormones are still in widespread and legal use, a continuing unwelcome chemical accompaniment to our meat.

The government—the FDA and other agencies—may have seemed slow in responding to the DES fiasco, but the government, like any leviathan, requires a long start-up to overcome initial inertia and develop momentum. All past and future victims of the DES fiasco can only hope that this momentum will not be lost.

# 8·DES and the Law

*"No question but it's [the DES lawsuits] the biggest case ever brought against the drug companies—and probably the biggest products liability case [sic] ever brought against American industry."*

ED HEAFY, *regional DES counsel for Eli Lilly and Company, as quoted by Connie Bruck ("Defense Lawyers Fight Over Strategy as Massive DES Battle Heats Up") in* The American Lawyer, *February 1979*

Although the medical problems engendered by DES are complex and far-reaching, the impact of this drug is by no means confined to health issues. DES has landed in the legal arena with all the potential of a hand grenade with its pin pulled.

The crux of the DES legal tangle is a principle of law known as liability. In a legal sense, liability has sweeping significance and includes nearly every kind of hazard or responsibility. An individual or corporation or government agency may be held liable—or accountable—for any debt, legal obligation, risk, or injury for which our laws ascribe responsibility. The law recognizes many categories of liability, such as personal liability, parental liability, employer's liability, and product liability. DES lawsuits involve the concept of product liability.

To understand why DES lawsuits have thus far been an uphill battle, it is helpful to know the grounds upon which product safety lawsuits may be based.

Basic to all product liability suits in which an unsafe product has caused an injury, the injured consumer must be prepared to prove three basic conditions of liability: (1) that the product was indeed defective; (2) that there was an injury; and (3) that the injury was caused by the defective product. If these three elements are proven, then the manufacturer of the unsafe product may be found liable and a cash award for damages may be given to the plaintiff, the person bringing the lawsuit.

Although this appears to be a simple procedure, and may indeed be quite straightforward in some cases, many other instances of product liability are not so clear and easy to prove. Then the concept of liability becomes bewilderingly varied and fraught with special conditions.

When a plaintiff brings legal suit against the manufacturer of a defective product that caused injury, the plaintiff's attorney must base the case on at least one of the following four grounds: (1) intentional tort (wrongdoing); (2) negligence; (3) breach of warranty; or (4) strict liability.

To illustrate each of these, consider the example of a lawn mower with a defective cutting blade. The consumer who has purchased this lawn mower takes it home and in the course of normal use, the mower blade catches a pebble. The blade, which is made of defective steel, snaps in two from the impact, sending a sharp metal fragment into the leg of the consumer, causing obvious pain and injury. The consumer files suit against the manufacturer because of a defective product, which caused injury during the course of normal use and anticipated wear and tear.

The attorney for the plaintiff will first establish the grounds for the lawsuit. If it can be shown that the lawn mower manufacturer was aware of the defect in the steel blade that snapped and did nothing to prevent it from going on the open market, the manufacturer may be sued on the basis of intentional tort or wrongdoing. If, however, the manufacturer was *not* aware of the defect because he did not perform adequate safety checking, the manufacturer may be sued for negligence. If the manufacturer took every reasonable precaution, but merely failed to warn the consumer that such an accident was possible, the manufacturer could be held liable on breach of warranty (that is, violation of the implied contract between the manufacturer and the consumer that the product was safe for the intended use).

Finally, even if the first three conditions do not apply—for example, if the manufacturer has taken the greatest care in designing and manufacturing the lawn mower, and has warned that accidents injurious to the user might still happen, the courts may *still* hold the manufacturer responsible for the injury under the concept of strict liability, which states that the manufacturer is liable for any and all defective or hazardous products, despite any and all precautions the manufacturer might have taken. The injured consumer may then be entitled to collect a cash award from the manufacturer to compensate him for lost wages, pain, and suffering.

A notable case in which the principle of strict liability was invoked involved the Ford Motor Company and one of its products, the Ford Mustang. In 1975 in Wisconsin, a Ford Mustang carrying four passengers was hit from behind, sending it out of control, whereupon it was hit a second time by another car. The second collision ruptured the gas tank of the Mustang, which exploded, killing two passengers and seriously burning the other two.

The families of the passengers sued Ford Motor Company, claiming the company should be held strictly liable for not recalling the 1967 Mustangs, which the company knew had faulty gas tanks that were apt to explode in a collision. (Under these alleged conditions, the company could also have been charged with intentional tort, negligence, and breach of warranty.) The Wisconsin State Supreme Court agreed with the plaintiffs and ruled against the Ford Motor Company, holding them strictly liable.

In prescription drug cases, strict liability is *not* applicable if the drug reasonably* appeared to be useful and desirable and reasonably safe at the time it was manufactured, and there

---

*Unreasonable*—As defined in law, an unreasonable risk is one where the product's risks outweigh its alleged benefits. For example, although rabies vaccine has the dangerous potential for causing the very disease it is designed to prevent, its risk is still considered reasonable by legal standards. Since untreated rabies will certainly cause hideous death, and the vaccine is the victim's only hope of survival, the risk inherent to the use of the vaccine is considered "reasonable."

was no medically recognizable risk that outweighed the drug's usefulness.

Once strict liability is made a basis for the lawsuit (it need not be the *only* basis), the plaintiff's attorney must determine *who* is liable (that is, *who* is to be sued). For example, if the driver of a car becomes involved in an accident injuring another person, the injured person may sue the driver. However, if someone other than the driver *owns* the car that caused the injury, the injured person may also sue the car owner if it can be proven that the driver had the car with its owner's permission. If, however, the driver stole the car, then the owner would not be held liable for the injuries caused by the driver.

Because identification of liable parties is not always clear-cut, the law contains a number of different conditions of liability to help define the liable parties. These include concert of action, alternative liability, and joint and several liability. DES litigation has added two new such concepts, namely, joint-enterprise or industry-wide liability, and market-share liability. Each of these concepts of liability defines the conditions under which a manufacturer may be held strictly liable.

*Concert of action.* To successfully sue based on the concept of concert of action, the plaintiff must prove that two or more parties (in the case of DES lawsuits these "parties" would be the drug companies) agreed, planned, and acted according to some common scheme which then causes injury. In concert of action, all participants in the scheme would bear equal responsibility.

The major legal difficulty for DES plaintiffs bringing suit based on concert of action is the fact that the drug companies did not act together (at the same time) in starting to manufacture DES; many of them came into and out of the DES market for varying reasons and at widely disparate intervals. So, it cannot be said that they acted according to a "common scheme."

*Alternative liability.* The theory of alternative liability may be applied in cases where more than one defendant acted wrong-fully, but only one defendant caused the plaintiff's injury and the plaintiff is unsure which defendant caused the injury. The burden of proof then switches to the defendants, and if one or more of them can prove innocence, then that defendant frees himself/itself from legal responsibility. In a DES lawsuit based on alternative liability, a drug company named in a lawsuit may be able to exculpate itself (clear itself of alleged fault) if it shows, for example, that it was not manufacturing DES at the time the plaintiff's mother took the drug.

Applied to DES litigation, the alternative liability theory appears at first to be appropriate and attractive, but as we shall see, it contains a major pitfall. The classic example of alternative liability involves two hunters who both simulta-neously shoot in the general direction of a third hunter. The third hunter is injured, but is unable to say which of the other two hunters shot him. It is clear that both hunters could have fired the shot that injured the third hunter, and unless one of the first two hunters can prove he did not fire the shot that caused injury, both are considered liable.

The law holds, then, that both wrongdoers should not be allowed to escape responsibility for the injury merely because the nature of the wrongdoing made it impossible for the plaintiff to identify the individual who actually inflicted the injury.

In the case of DES, however, there were not two, but hundreds of defendants, so that most drug companies named in any given lawsuit are most probably *not* responsible for having manufactured the DES pills responsible for the injuries in question. Attorneys for the defendant-drug companies would argue that to place liability on all DES manufacturers under these circumstances would be an unfair burden.

*Joint and several liability.* The concept of joint and several liability also appears to be appropriate to DES litigation and indeed has been partially used to formulate the newer theory of joint enterprise or industry-wide liability.

A liability is said to be joint and several when a plaintiff may sue one or more or all the defendants named in a suit, so that each defendant is liable for the entire amount of the liability if the plaintiff chooses not to pursue any of the other defendants.

For example, if three people cosign a loan note, then upon default on the payment, the loan institution can hold all the cosigners jointly responsible. But, if two of the cosigners declare bankruptcy, the loan institution may hold the third person alone responsible for the entire debt. The third person is then said to be severally responsible.

Applied to DES, this concept is weak because it requires the identification of the defendants, something that is impossible in most DES cases.

*Joint enterprise or industry-wide liability.* Because none of the established bases of liability have prevailed in courtrooms so far as applied to DES lawsuits, plaintiffs' attorneys and the California Supreme Court evolved a new theory of liability, which combines some of the elements of each of the more established descriptions, including alternative liability, concert of action, and joint and several liability.

Joint-enterprise or industry-wide liability holds that all the drug companies that manufactured DES for prescription to pregnant women are similarly liable for injuries caused by DES because all drug companies adhered to an industry-wide standard of safety and an identical formula. Joint-enterprise liability would apply only in those cases where the plaintiff could not identify the specific drug company which manufactured the DES in her case.

The DES plaintiff would then have to prove the following points for a successful suit. That:

1. All the defendants manufactured a generically identical product.

2. The plaintiff could not reasonably be expected to identify the brand of the product causing her injury.

3. The plaintiff's injury resulted from the defendant's product, or from a product exactly like the defendant's.

4. The defendants had a legal responsibility to provide a safe product to the plaintiff and others like her.

5. There is "clear and convincing evidence" that probably one of the named defendants manufactured the injurious product. In the case of DES, this would mean that the drug companies named as defendants had a large enough share of the DES market that any one of them could likely have manufactured the DES taken by the DES mother in the case.

6. All of the 267 manufacturers of DES adhered to an equally inadequate standard of safety in manufacturing the drug.

7. All defendants fulfill the criteria of the specifically proposed cause of action, whether that cause be negligence, breach of warranty, or strict liability.

Currently, there are more than 1,000 DES cases as of this writing pending in nearly every state in the country, in various stages of litigation. Of those that have already been tried, only four have been decided in favor of the DES daughter-plaintiff, and of those four, one was reversed by a higher court.

What this illustrates is that DES daughters wishing to sue because of their DES exposure will almost surely be in for a long, hard legal battle.

In this age, when billions of dollars worth of millions of manufactured items are sold every year, any legal decision that places greater responsibility upon manufacturers to produce safe goods has a potentially enormous financial impact upon both the manufacturers and their insurance companies.

In Wisconsin, for example, where product liability laws that are largely favorable to the consumer have been established, manufacturers and their insurance companies are becoming alarmed. In February 1981, a coalition of manufacturers, corporate lawyers, and insurance companies formed a group to combat Wisconsin's liberal product liability laws by initiating restrictive legislation. The group, which calls itself the Wisconsin Task Force for Product Liability Reform, plans to introduce to the state legislature four bills that would place statutory controls on product liability lawsuits. They claim that liability insurance rates are "sky-rocketing" as a result of the increased number of mega-dollar awards to injured consumers.

Consumer advocates feel otherwise. They maintain that such awards to injured consumers still constitute only a small fraction of the amount of money insurance companies collect in the form of insurance payments from manufacturers. Product liability litigator Robert Habush, a Wisconsin attorney, says that anticonsumer statutes like those being written by the Product Liability Task Force simply reflect the efforts of those groups that have the "most to lose because of sloppy manufacturing and hazardous products."

One of the statutory limitations the task force wishes to impose is a 10-year limitation on product safety lawsuits, a law that would bar consumers from suing for damages resulting from a defective product after 10 years from the time the product was released for sale. Such a regulation, for example, would automatically bar suits involving DES.

Statutes of limitations, proving injury, and identifying the defendant are three of the major legal hurdles DES plaintiffs have had to overcome to win a lawsuit.

*Statute of limitations.* Most states specify a period of time, ranging anywhere from two to 20 years from the time a product was sold, after which a person may not file suit for an injury caused by that product. Although fairly straightforward in most instances, a statute of limitations is patently unfair in those cases involving DES or any product that causes injury many years after exposure to the product. How strictly interpreted and applied the statute of limitations is in any given place varies from state to state, and even from judge to judge.

For example, in a 1979 lawsuit brought by a DES daughter against E. R. Squibb & Sons, a Florida judge in effect threw the case out of court by hewing to a strict interpretation of

Florida's statute of limitations, which bars product liability suits after 12 years from the date of delivery of the product to its original purchaser, regardless of the date the defect was or should have been discovered.

In contrast, the Illinois court held that the two-year state statute of limitations did not bar the lawsuit of Anne Needham, who was suing White Laboratories, because there was no possible way Ms. Needham could have known within two years of her DES exposure of the DES-caused cancer she would develop.

*Proving injury.* As stated in chapters 3 and 4, while most DES daughters have benign genital tract abnormalities as a result of their DES exposure, a relatively small percentage of them develop DES-related cancer. There have been a number of lawsuits initiated by daughters with benign abnormalities based on the complaint that as a result of their DES exposure, they have an increased *risk* for cancer.

The first class-action lawsuit in behalf of DES daughters was filed in 1974 by attorney Paul Rheingold, naming his own daughter as plaintiff in a suit against 20 drug companies. "The judge threw the case out of court on the ground that Rheingold was not claiming his daughter was injured, just DES-exposed, and without current injury there could be no suit," wrote Connie Bruck in her article about drug company lawyer strategies in the February 1979 issue of *The American Lawyer.*

The lesson to be learned from this decision is that a DES daughter must prove she suffered DES-caused *injury* to successfully wage a product liability suit. And, the simple truth is that current medical opinion holds that the benign changes found in most DES daughters are *abnormalities*, not *injuries*. A similar opinion was rendered by an Illinois court in ruling against former U.S. Senator Patsy Mink (a DES mother) and her coplaintiffs because the plaintiffs did not demonstrate injury.

So far in DES lawsuits, cancer has been the only DES-caused condition legally recognized as an injury. The concept of DES-caused injury may be broadened, however, if—in the future—DES daughters *and* sons start suing because of DES-caused infertility.

## • WHO'S RESPONSIBLE? IDENTIFYING THE DEFENDANT

The most significant legal stumbling block for DES daughters suing on the basis of DES-caused injuries has been to determine *who* is responsible, or in other words, who is the appropriate party to sue.

There have been four suggested targets for DES lawsuits— (1) physicians who prescribed DES; (2) pharmacists who dispensed DES; (3) the government (specifically, the Food and Drug Administration) which approved DES; and (4) most important of all, the drug companies that manufactured and marketed DES.

*Physicians as defendants.* To date, few DES plaintiffs have targeted physicians in their lawsuits, although many DES-prescribing physicians remain fearful of lawsuits.

One reason for this is that physicians are *not* expected to be the final authorities on the effectiveness and safety of drugs. It is generally accepted that the physician may reasonably rely on the drug manufacturers to provide the medical profession with information about a drug. This is the case; the vast majority of physicians do get their information about drugs from the drug companies—either through drug company sales representatives or from drug company literature.

A second reason is that to successfully sue a physician, a plaintiff would have to prove malpractice, and a generally accepted legal tenet is that a physician should not be held liable for engaging in medical practices that were generally accepted at the time the physician practiced them, even though superseding scientific knowledge reveals those older practices to be faulty.

*Pharmacists as defendants.* In 1977, when Joyce Bichler made her first and unsuccessful attempt to recover damages for her DES-caused cancer, her suit named three defendants—a physician, a drug manufacturer, and her mother's pharmacist. In ruling against the suit, the court stated that the pharmacist could not be held liable because he did nothing to alter the product, DES, as it came from the manufacturer, nor did he make any express claims about its safety. Finally, the court stated that when purchasing a prescription drug, the consumer relies on the physician's judgement and not on the pharmacist's judgement as to the suitability of the drug. (And, as mentioned above, the physician relies on the drug company!)

*The Food and Drug Administration as the defendant.* In 1978, in *Gray versus the United States,* a DES daughter from Texas sued the federal government in the person of the Food and Drug Administration for failing to adequately test DES, for approving it for use, and for representing it as safe. The court ruled against Ms. Gray on the grounds that certain "discretionary functions" of government officials involving policy judgements and the "balancing of a risk-benefit formula" are exempt from legal liability under the Federal Tort Claims Act. The court held that the FDA's actions with respect to DES fell into this category, making this agency immune to Ms. Gray's suit.

*Drug manufacturers as defendants.* From a legal standpoint, by far the most logical defendants in DES litigation are the pharmaceutical companies that manufactured DES, for drug companies are held to the standard of being the experts where drugs are concerned.

However, despite the obvious nature of their responsibilities to the consumer, as far as DES has been concerned, suing drug companies has also proven difficult. The major reason for this is that the vast majority of DES mothers and daughters have no idea *which* of the 267 DES manufacturers made the specific pills which they, the plaintiffs, were exposed to. A brief history of drug company involvement with DES helps explain why this is so.

In 1938, when British biochemist E. C. Dodds developed

DES, he did not patent the drug. This left the formula available for any drug company to use. Within two years, 12 companies had filed 12 separate applications with the Food and Drug Administration for approval to manufacture and market DES. In December 1940, FDA officials decided to pool all the clinical data on DES into a single "master file." To insure that the chemical characteristics of each company's product was identical, the FDA also instructed the applicant drug companies to use the same United States Pharmacopoeia standard. And, further, the FDA similarly standardized the literature and product labeling for all DES. Because of this industry-wide standardization of this one drug, DES was often marketed under its generic names—diethylstilbestrol, stilbestrol, or simply, DES. (There were also numerous brand names, which are listed in the appendix.)

So, that while many women knew they were receiving DES, there was often no identifying brand name to remember, nor was it reasonable to expect that women might keep a sample of pills or a pill container to offer as proof in court perhaps two decades after the pills were prescribed.

Because the imposition of legal liability generally depends on the plaintiff being able to identify the party that caused the injury, DES lawsuits seemed doomed to failure from the start. Doomed to failure, that is, until July 16, 1979.

### • THE CASES

*Joyce Bichler and joint-enterprise liability.* On the afternoon of that summer day in 1979, a six-person, Bronx, New York, jury awarded half a million dollars to Joyce Bichler, a 25-year-old DES daughter who had lost her vagina, uterus, and one ovary to DES-caused cancer.

Her attorneys had based her case on the novel legal theory of "joint-enterprise liability," claiming that although Ms.

Bichler and her mother did not know the identity of the drug company that manufactured the specific pills Mrs. Bichler took, Joyce Bichler was still entitled to collect from Eli Lilly and Co. (the single, largest DES manufacturer) because all manufacturers of DES adhered to common standards and manufactured an identically defective product. The Bichler attorneys targeted Eli Lilly and Co. because it was among the first and largest producers of DES, manufacturing an estimated 40 percent of all DES.

Lilly's attorneys appealed the decision to the Appellate division of the New York State Supreme Court and one and one-half years later, in February 1981, that court unanimously reaffirmed the decision of the Bronx jury.

The Bichler decision is a landmark one. By accepting the novel legal argument of joint-enterprise liability, the New York courts stretched the legally accepted boundaries of all products liability cases and placed upon all manufacturers a more exacting measure of responsibility to the consumer than had been the case up to the Bichler decision. As Joyce Bichler said following her legal victory, "I never did this for myself. I did it for every consumer. They [the manufacturers] can't use us as guinea pigs."

The Bichler decision also paves the way for hundreds more DES cases across the country where the particular manufacturer of the DES pills taken is unknown.

*The Judith Sindell decision and market share liability.* On March 20, 1980—after the Bronx jury decided in favor of Joyce Bichler, but before the New York Supreme Court considered the appeal in that case—the California Supreme Court added a new dimension to DES litigation, as well as to products liability law in general.

Judith Sindell, a DES daughter who had developed bladder cancer as a result of her DES exposure, also did not know which drug company manufactured the DES her mother had taken. Still, in her suit she named Abbot Laboratories and four other drug companies on a legal basis similar to that used in the Bichler case. Sindell's attorneys held that regardless of which particular brand of DES Ms. Sindell's mother took, the defendants were jointly liable (the five defendants in this suit purportedly produced 90 percent of all the DES) because they relied upon each other's tests of the drug and adhered to an industry-wide safety standard which, as it turned out, was inadequate.

In rendering a decision in favor of Ms. Sindell, the judge gave the plaintiff and others like her the right to sue drug companies even though they could not identify the manufacturer of the pills that injured them.

The judge reasoned that "advances in science and technology create fungible [interchangeable] goods which may harm consumers and which cannot be traced to any specific producer." In addition, the judge wrote in his decision that the conduct of the drug companies in marketing a drug whose effects "are delayed for many years played a significant role in creating unavailability of proof."

But, because there were hundreds of companies that manufactured DES for pregnancy problems, the judge stated that it would be unfair to apply the classic concept of alternative liability in which there is a limited number of wrongdoers among which one wrongdoer is most certainly the one who caused the injury at issue. Targeting just one or even several drug companies out of the 267 that produced DES would still allow a substantial chance, said the judge, that the drug company that actually produced the injury at issue would escape punishment.

To insure then that liability for DES-caused injury was as fairly apportioned as possible, the California Supreme Court developed a new theory of liability called "market-share liability," which is rooted in "industry-wide liability" (a more appropriate name, said the judge, than enterprise liability). Applied to the manufacturers of DES, market-share liability calls for the defendant drug companies to share in the cost of damages to an injured plaintiff according to their percentage of the whole DES market.

The drug companies, of course, appealed the decision of the California Supreme Court, but in the fall of 1980, the United States Supreme Court refused to hear the case, which effectively reaffirms the California court's decision. Another landmark victory for DES victims!

*Anne Needham and the technical error.* If ever there was a "sure bet" DES lawsuit, Anne Needham's was it. Ms. Needham was 20 years old when she, like Joyce Bichler, underwent a hysterectomy and vaginectomy for DES-caused vaginal cancer. However, unlike Ms. Bichler, Ms. Needham was able to name the drug company that manufactured the pills her mother took; her own father had been the pharmacist who had filled her mother's DES prescriptions.

The case was a straightforward example of negligence and strict liability. Anne Needham's attorney argued that the dienestrol (a DES-type artificial estrogen) Mrs. Needham took caused Anne's cancer, that White Laboratories, which manufactured the drug knew or should have known the drug could cause cancer, and so should be held liable for the injury the drug subsequently caused Anne. The Chicago jury returned a verdict in favor of Anne Needham and awarded her $800,000. That was in August 1979.

White Laboratories appealed and on January 27, 1981, the United States Court of Appeals for the Seventh Circuit reversed the decision of the Chicago jury. The reversal came as a stunning surprise to everyone interested in the success of DES litigation.

The reason for the reversal was as aggravating as the reversal itself, boiling down to erroneous instructions given by the judge to the Chicago jury. When the jury was ready to consider the case, after all the evidence and testimony had been given, the judge had instructed the jury that they could find White Laboratories liable on either of two grounds: (1) that White Laboratories knew or should have known that dienestrol could cause cancer, or (2) (and this was the judge's erroneous charge to the jury) that the product was unavoidably dangerous and the benefits didn't outweigh the risk. It was this second ground that was to prove the undoing of the jury verdict. The jury, of course, brought in a verdict for the plaintiff, but never was asked to specify which of the two grounds it had based its decision on. Since White Laboratories had never presented a defense on the second charge, this was an erroneous basis upon which to find White guilty. So, technically, the jury's decision, which may have been based on the second ground, had to be reversed, and a new trial ordered. Anne Needham and her attorney must now go through the entire courtroom procedure all over again, all because of a procedural error.

Although—based on the Sindell decision and the two courtroom victories for Joyce Bichler—there are grounds for believing that DES plaintiffs will eventually emerge victorious in the courtroom, what the cited cases demonstrate are the many legal pitfalls that exist for DES litigants and the arduous but necessary restructuring of established legal theories that has already begun.

## The Cost of the DES Lawsuits

Without even considering jury awards to DES daughters, or out-of-court settlements between drug companies and plaintiffs, DES has already cost a fortune to litigate.

For example, according to Connie Bruck writing in *The American Lawyer,* in a case brought by plaintiff's attorney, Herbert Kolsby of Philadelphia against E. R. Squibb & Sons, it cost Mr. Kolsby $60,000 "just to bring the case to trial, not counting all the hours of his office time." (In personal injury cases, it is customary for plaintiff's attorneys not to charge their clients a fee *per se,* but rather to take an agreed-upon percentage of a cash award or settlement. So, the cost of legal research, filing formal papers, and so on, is paid by the attorney.) Although this case was eventually won by Squibb, it cost the drug company—or more correctly, the drug company's insurance company—a quarter of a million dollars for legal defense.

But, especially with the Sindell and Bichler victories, it is the potential for hundreds of successful lawsuits against them that is unnerving the drug companies. Personal damages awards in both the Bichler and Needham cases (the reversal of the Needham case notwithstanding) were $500,000 to more than $750,000 each.

So far, well over 400 DES daughters have developed cancer. If all of them sue and win damages similar to those awarded in the Bichler and Needham cases, it would cost the drug companies close to $300 million for awards alone, not even counting legal defense costs. That does not include the distinct possibility that as time passes and inflation continues to rise, the amount of these awards and settlements could go even higher.

Nor do these figures take into account the many DES daughters who have sustained DES-caused injuries other than cancer, such as the inability to bear children and who may sue. Then, we are talking about thousands more potential plaintiffs, and the cost to the drug companies could sky-rocket.

Nor do these figures take into account the fact that DES sons have not yet entered the legal arena. It may well eventually be shown that DES sons have developed testicular or prostate cancers as a result of their exposure; it has already been shown that many of these men are sterile because they were exposed *in utero* to DES. What happens if these men begin filing suit against the drug companies? Then the number of potential DES litigants might well double!

Eli Lilly and Co. claims its total sales for DES prescribed for pregnancy were roughly $2.5 million. They are currently being sued for about $4 billion. It's a sure bet that Lilly would gladly return every penny of its DES profits if it would somehow erase the whole miserable, expensive business.

## The Overall Impact of the DES Lawsuits

Astronomical as they may seem, even these costs may well be just for openers. The new theories of joint-enterprise liability (or industry-wide liability) and market-share liability are serious legal events for many more industries than just the drug companies.

Market-share and joint-enterprise liability will be applicable in *any* cases of personal injury when it is impossible to identify the manufacturer of the product causing the injury. For example, under these new theories, people may sue who have been injured by chemical pollutants, or radioactive wastes, or asbestos, or drugs, all of which cause injuries that do not become evident until many years after exposure and in all cases of which it would be impossible to identify the precise manufacturer.

DES has stretched the legal limits of product liability in such a significant way that *all* manufacturers must now hold their products to the highest possible standards of safety and effectiveness—or run the risk of being sued out of existence.

## • ALTERNATIVES TO LITIGATION

*What about a drug company DES fund?* Many people have suggested that the drug companies should initiate and finance a DES fund that would pay for the cost of the semiannual examinations all DES daughters must undergo, as well as any necessary medical treatment.

Such a plan was actually discussed in 1976 between drug companies and DES plaintiffs' attorneys, with Eli Lilly and Co. among the participants.

The plan was to identify all the DES daughters in the country and then make small cash settlements with them to help defray the cost of medical care. However, these preliminary talks soon dissolved as the cost of such a plan became apparent. Even if $10,000 were awarded to each of the minimum one million DES daughters with adenosis—and $10,000 is considered small by today's litigation standards—it would cost the drug industry $10 billion just at the outset. By comparison, the estimated $140 million settlement paid to thalidomide victims by West German drug manufacturers seems paltry.

There are no new plans to establish a DES fund, and the drug companies seem to have decided to take their chances in court. Perhaps they may eventually regret that decision, but the way it looks now, they are between the proverbial "rock and a hard place."

*Legislation.* Legislation to identify and provide medical services for DES daughters has been somewhat more successful than the DES fund, but is still far from comprehensive.

So far, three states—New York, Illinois, and California—have enacted legislation *and* appropriated special state funds to launch a public information campaign about DES, offer free DES screening clinics, and establish a plan to protect the DES-exposed from insurance discrimination. Maine has passed similar legislation but without an appropriation of special funds; however, it is paying for the programs mandated by its legislature through regular operating capital.

Maryland, Michigan, and Massachusetts have DES legislation pending as of this writing; New Jersey's bill was vetoed by the governor because of budget considerations; and Oregon passed a resolution to encourage the identification and medical screening of the DES-exposed in that state. While a resolution is the least effective step a law-making body can take, it is, at the least, a recognition of the problem.

## • PRACTICAL LEGAL ADVICE FOR THE DES-EXPOSED

(The following information has been taken from advice published by the Coalition for the Medical Rights of Women in San Francisco. Their publication is titled, "Your Legal Rights in Health Care.")

You have a legal right to competent, safe, and effective health care. If you are injured because of defective or unsafe products or through incompetent medical practices, you may sue. The money you may recover through such legal remedies cannot restore you or a loved one to a previously healthy condition, but it can help you to recover lost wages and medical expenses, as well as compensate you for pain and suffering.

*When should you seek the advice of a lawyer?* If you believe you have been injured as a result of your DES exposure, consult a lawyer who will help you determine whether or not you have a case. Don't fail to act because you think too much time has passed or that you must bear the consequences of having agreed to use the product and treatment.

*How to find the right attorney.* Since product liability and medical negligence cases such as DES require special technical knowledge and experience, not all attorneys will be competent to handle a DES case. For the names of attorneys who have experience handling DES cases, contact either the New York or San Francisco office of DES Action (addresses in appendix), or write to the American Trial Lawyers' Association, 1050 31st St., N.W., Washington, D.C. 20007, for a list of attorneys in your area who are experienced in products liability and medical negligence cases.

*How much will an attorney cost you?* An ethical products liability and medical negligence attorney will work on a contingency basis. This means that there is no charge to the plaintiff unless you win your case or settle out of court for an agreed-upon amount of money. Then your lawyer will take 33 percent to 45 percent of the award or settlement as the legal fee.

*Working with your attorney.* Once you have decided to file suit, your lawyer should tell you the strengths and weaknesses of your case. Before you go to trial, your opponent may offer to settle your case out of court. The settlement offer is usually less than what your attorney would ask for at trial, but this must be weighed by your lawyer and you against the risks and expenses of a trial. For example, in a trial you may lose and get nothing, or you may win but receive less than the settlement offer, or you may win the same amount as the offer or more.

Suing is not the answer for every DES-exposed person. It takes a great toll in money, time, and intellectual and emotional energy. But, if you and your attorney remain convinced that a legal remedy is appropriate to your situation, then remember, it has been done successfully, and it can be done again.

# 9·The Drugs Pregnant Women Still Take

*"What has happened will happen again,*
*What has been done we still must do,*
*Nothing under the sun is entirely new."*
                                    *Ecclesiastes, 1:9*

Early in 1980, a small article appeared in one of the women's magazines heralding the development of a group of experimental drugs that could prevent premature births by inhibiting uterine contractions. The drugs belonged to a group of chemicals called beta-sympathomimetics. The article expressed hope that one of the drugs, ritodrine, might soon be approved for clinical use by the Food and Drug Administration.

Forty years after DES was approved for clinical use, and nine years after the DES cancer connection was established, the siren call of another "easy answer" to pregnancy problems was being sounded once again.

Although it is unfair to compare ritodrine and its sister drugs with DES (the beta-sympathomimetics are *not* hormones and have entirely different effects on the body from that of DES), what *is* fair to question is the advocacy of *any* drug treatment during pregnancy.

A quick run through of any drug directory will reveal that the vast majority of drugs are contraindicated for use during pregnancy. The reason for this is compelling. Any substance that a pregnant woman puts into her body—whether it be the caffeine in a cup of coffee, the alcohol in a martini, or the cannabis in a joint of marijuana—she also puts in the developing fetal body inside her womb.

The placenta—a disk-shaped piece of tissue connecting the fetus to its mother—was once thought of as a protective barrier for the fetus. It is now known to permit the passage into the fetal circulation of virtually every substance found in the mother's bloodstream. And, the exquisitely sensitive fetal tissue, primed by nature to react to many kinds of biochemical stimuli in order to develop and mature, also reacts to other chemical stimuli.

So, for example, thalidomide will inhibit the development of arms and legs; alcohol will cause fetal alcohol syndrome; and DES causes genital tract abnormalities and possibly vaginal cancer years later.

In spite of the fact that we have been made tragically aware that *any* drug a pregnant woman takes can potentially harm her unborn child, many physicians, as well as many patients, are still seduced by the prepackaged, premeasured, sterilized, laboratory-tested promises of pills and injections purporting to alleviate pregnancy problems.

## • PREMATURE LABOR AND BIRTH

To understand why a drug like ritodrine was developed, let us sidetrack for a bit to consider why premature birth is so undesirable.

About 8 percent of all pregnancies in the United States terminate in premature labor and birth. That means that eight out of every 100 pregnant women go into labor sometime after the fifteenth week of pregnancy, but before the pregnancy has reached its full term of roughly 40 weeks. If birth occurs much before the thirty-sixth week, or ninth month, of pregnancy, the baby might be too small to survive on its own, outside the womb.

A baby that weighs less than $5\frac{1}{2}$ pounds (2,500 grams) is considered low birth weight, and is 20 times more likely to be sick or dangerously underdeveloped at birth than its full-term brothers and sisters. An infant weighing 1,000 grams or less at birth has its chances of survival reduced to a mere 30 percent, and of those who *do* survive—according to one study appearing in the journal *Pediatrics*—one-third have significant physical and/or mental defects.

It is during the last trimester of pregnancy that the fetus gains most of its weight and matures sufficiently to thrive on its own once it is born. At 5½ months of pregnancy, for example, the fetus weighs only about one pound; by seven months, it weighs roughly three pounds; by the eighth month, four and one-half pounds, and by birth, six and one-half to seven pounds.

It is obvious, then, that the closer to term a baby is born, the better its chances for surviving *and* the better its chances for maturing sufficiently *in utero* to be healthy at birth.

About half of all cases of premature labor can be accounted for by a variety of predisposing factors, such as premature rupture of the membranes, incompetent cervix, uterine overdistension (as in multiple births), and an abnormally small or hypoplastic uterus. In DES daughters, an abnormally small uterus has been cited unofficially by a number of doctors as the cause of mid- or late-pregnancy miscarriages. The constricted, T-shaped uterus (*see* chapter 4) characteristic of many DES daughters may simply be unable to stretch sufficiently to accommodate a rapidly growing, third-trimester fetus.

In the other half of premature labor cases, no one knows the cause. However, *that* it happens is of grave concern. In addition to the high rates of illness and death among "preemies," premature labor and delivery are costly in terms of dollars. One author, writing in the *American Journal of Obstetrics and Gynecology* in August 1980, estimated the average cost of medical care for a premature infant who eventually survives ranges from $64,000 to $140,000.

So, it is easy to understand—in terms of death, of disability, and of dollars—why doctors are anxious to find an effective means of delaying the birth of infants whose mothers go into labor before term.

Toward this end, doctors have used a variety of treatments. The first, the simplest, the cheapest, and the most obvious of these is the surprisingly effective "treatment" of complete bed rest. According to a *Quick Reference to OB-GYN Procedures* (second edition), about 70 percent of cases in several studies of premature uterine contractions responded to bed rest alone.

However, if rhythmic contractions persist and the woman and her pregnancy meet certain medical criteria, doctors may initiate more active treatment.

These criteria include the following. The doctor must ascertain that the woman really is in premature labor (that is, rhythmic contractions persisting even after a course of bed rest), that cervical dilation is beginning, that the fetus is normal and healthy, that there are no reasons *not* to prolong pregnancy (see list below), that the membranous sack surrounding the fetus is intact, that there is no bleeding, and that the labor is sufficiently premature to warrant active medical treatment. (This generally means that the estimated weight of the fetus is under $5\frac{1}{2}$ pounds, or the pregnancy is fewer than 35 weeks advanced.)

In addition, drugs to stop uterine contractions should *not* be used if the mother is hemorrhaging or her membranes have been ruptured, or if she has high blood pressure, diabetes, eclampsia or pre-eclampsia (a condition occurring in pregnancy characterized, among other things, by uncontrolled high blood pressure, and which can be fatal to mother and baby). Nor should contraction-inhibiting drugs be given if the mother has preexisting heart disease, hyperthyroidism, or a cervix dilated more than five centimeters. Drugs should also be withheld if the fetus is dead or malformed, or if it is suffering from intrauterine growth retardation (a condition in which the fetus fails to thrive and develop inside the womb; in this case, the baby, even premature, might fare better in a newborn intensive care facility than inside its mother's womb).

*Alcohol.* Alcohol, specifically ethanol, has been among the earlier drugs used to stop premature contractions. A solution of ethanol and water is dripped intravenously into the pregnant woman over a period of 12 hours, in much the same manner as a transfusion. The dose of alcohol is gradually tapered off, and then stopped. Various studies have shown that ethanol is not a great deal more successful in stopping labor, according to *A Quick Reference to OB-GYN Procedures,* than total bed rest.

In addition, this treatment is psychoactive; it adversely affects the patient's behavior and ability to think. In a word, it makes her drunk. It also causes headaches, nausea, vomiting, and the risk that the patient will choke by breathing in her own vomit. The alcohol is also dangerous to the fetus since it passes freely through the placenta and into the fetal circulation. For these reasons, and because other drugs have become available for treating premature labor, ethanol is losing favor.

*The anti-prostaglandins.* Prostaglandins are substances found in tissues throughout the body which, among other things, affect muscle tone and help cause uterine contractions. Anti-prostaglandins work to stop uterine contractions by preventing the body from producing prostaglandins. Anti-prostaglandins are administered to pregnant women in the same transfusion-like manner as ethanol.

In addition to common aspirin, which has a mild anti-prostaglandin effect but which can provoke bleeding in a threatened pregnancy, two other anti-prostaglandin drugs have been frequently used in patients with premature labor, although neither has been approved specifically for this use. These drugs are indomethacin and naproxen.

Although both these drugs are effective in inhibiting uterine contractions, they also have some highly undesirable side effects. They both freely cross the placenta and enter the fetal circulation. Once there, they affect the blood-clotting mechanisms of the fetus (not unlike aspirin), and production of the infant's own prostaglandins and hence, fetal muscle tone. But, most seriously, they have the potential for prematurely closing the ductus arteriosus.* If this duct closes before the infant is born, blood will be unable to travel back to the placenta for oxygen, and the infant can die or be severely damaged because of oxygen deprivation.

The result, then, of using naproxen or indomethacin, is an unacceptable risk for the unborn infant. In a review of both these drugs, the editors of *Obstetrical and Gynecological Survey* wrote that "it appears that the use of naproxen or indomethacin for the arrest of uterine contractions of premature labor is contraindicated because of the possible adverse effects on fetal and neonatal cardiopulmonary physiology."

*The beta-sympathomimetics.* The third group of drugs—after alcohol and the anti-prostaglandins—is the one to which the recently approved ritodrine belongs. These are called beta-sympathomimetics because they mimic the action of the body's own sympathetic nervous system which, among other things, causes the uterine musculature to stop contracting.

There have been several beta-sympathomimetics on the market for a number of years, used to treat, among other conditions, chronic bronchitis and asthma. These drugs are salbutamol (albuterol), isoxsuprine, and terbutaline. All three have been used to inhibit the contractions of premature labor, with a fair degree of success. However, these drugs can cause discomfort—sometimes reaching considerable levels—in the mother, as well as some measurable side effects in the fetus.

Initial treatment for premature labor consists of administering a beta-sympathomimetic by intravenous drip over a period of 24 hours, by which time uterine contractions have

---

*Because the lungs of the fetus are nonfunctional, the fetal heart has a special anatomic structure called the *ductus arteriosus* (an arterial duct), which shunts oxygen-depleted blood away from the nonfunctional lungs and down to the placenta where it picks up oxygen and is recirculated. Under normal conditions, the ductus arteriosus closes instantaneously at birth, as soon as the baby draws its first breath. The closing of this duct at that moment sends the baby's oxygen-depleted blood to the newly functioning lungs for re-oxygenation, the system that remains for the life of the individual.

generally ceased. The intravenous drip is then followed by oral doses of the same drug in pill form for days, weeks, or sometimes months, depending upon how much longer the pregnancy has to go. The side effects of these drugs, when given intravenously, include nausea, vomiting, headaches, diarrhea, changes in blood pressure, and an abnormally rapid heartbeat.

Ritodrine, the most thoroughly investigated of the beta-sympathomimetics and the *only* one to be approved for use specifically to inhibit premature uterine contractions, has side effects similar to those of its sister compounds. In addition to the effects just cited, these compounds (ritodrine included) cross the placenta and enter the fetal circulation, causing the fetal heart to beat abnormally fast. Still, extensive testing of ritodrine has indicated the drug is relatively safe and effective. So far, it has been found that even babies whose heartbeats rose to 160 beats per minute while they were exposed *in utero* to the drug, were born in good condition, following a drug-induced prolongation of pregnancy.

Although the side effects of ritodrine are reportedly less severe than those of the other beta-sympathomimetics, as of this writing we should note that there has been only a two-year follow-up of human babies exposed *in utero* to this drug. So, we still do not know the long-term effects—if any—of this drug.

Still, a great many skilled and conscientious doctors are glad to have ritodrine approved and available. Dr. Philip Farrell, professor of pediatrics at the University of Wisconsin and a nationally recognized perinatologist (an expert in the care of infants during the period of late pregnancy and just after birth), said of ritodrine, "For better or for worse, I'm happy they've approved it." Dr. Farrell went on to point out that even though the drug has some undesirable side effects and possibly (although not necessarily probably) some unknown long-range ill effects, he explained that the drug allows doctors to "buy" enough time for the developing fetus to give it a chance for some possibly life-saving maturing inside the mother's womb.

"Prematurity," says Dr. Farrell, "is still the major problem of newborns." And the biggest complication of prematurity, says Dr. Farrell, is immature lungs, which lead to respiratory distress syndrome, an often fatal condition of premature or low-birth-weight infants. Because a fetus gains as much as 25 grams per day during the last three months of pregnancy, and because this additional weight is accompanied by a parallel development of the lungs, each day that the fetus remains inside the mother's womb gives it a better chance of survival.

When ritodrine is administered in conjunction with certain kinds of steroids that hasten lung development, then ritodrine, says Dr. Farrell, can prolong pregnancy sufficiently to make the difference between a healthy baby or a sick one with lung disease that may necessitate months of intensive medical attention. He says that if ritodrine can delay birth by even as little as 72 hours, steroids can often speed up the maturing process of the lungs enough to make a big difference.

However, there is a caveat to this dual treatment. A few women who have received ritodrine and steroids simultaneously have developed pulmonary edema, a condition in which excess fluid accumulates in the tissue of the lungs, and in severe cases, could lead to heart failure.

Although ritodrine may be a useful drug if given judiciously by experts such as Dr. Farrell, who works in conjunction with high-risk obstetrical specialists, the potential for overuse and misuse of this drug looms large. There are always pregnant women. There are always problem pregnancies. And, these problems are always traumatic events for both mother-to-be and her physician who is expected to keep both mother and infant alive and healthy.

The siren call of an "easy" solution to at least one common pregnancy problem—premature labor—will seduce many. If we have learned anything from the DES episode, it is that doctors with little or no experience in managing high-risk pregnancies will not hesitate to prescribe a drug if that drug is readily available and if popular medical scuttlebutt has it that the drug is an easy answer to a tough and emotional problem and if the drug company sales representatives are convincing enough.

Remember, that while there is no evidence so far that ritodrine will cause long-term harm to mother and child, there is simply not enough long-term experience with it to prove that it *won't* cause harm. For this reason, it should be used only by specialists and *only according to the most stringent criteria.*

## • GENERAL ADVICE TO PREGNANT WOMEN ABOUT DRUGS

If a pregnant woman is basically healthy, she should stay away from drugs!

The message is so simple and the evidence of harm from drugs taken during pregnancy so obvious, one would think all pregnant women would *know* by now that they should not take drugs unless there is a superseding medical reason that dictates otherwise. But many pregnant women don't heed the warnings. It seems that each new generation of pregnant women must learn for itself that drugs can harm their unborn children. For example, a 1979 University of Florida study of 168 pregnant women found that these women used an astounding average of 11 drugs—both prescription and over-the-counter—per pregnancy!

Tranquilizers to quell nausea in early pregnancy are still a popular item, in spite of the thalidomide tragedy. However, Bendectin, a widely prescribed morning-sickness drug, has been associated with an increase in birth defects. In 1978, 3.4 million prescriptions of Bendectin were written in this country, and earned revenues for its manufacturer, Richardson-Merrell, Inc., of $14.4 million. In 1980, Richardson-Merrell was successfully sued by a Florida family whose Bendectin baby had been born with hand and chest deformities. In the fall of 1980, the FDA convened a panel to examine the pros and cons of Bendectin as a morning-sickness drug, and preliminary evidence has indicated that Bendectin might, indeed, cause deformities in the young fetus.

The lesson from this is that while the nausea of pregnancy might be uncomfortable, or even distressing, it may well be safer than the relief offered by drugs.

The evidence against using drugs during pregnancy extends even to the "social" drugs—alcohol, caffeine, and cigarettes. Women who drink heavily or even just regularly during pregnancy run the risk of producing children with fetal alcohol syndrome. These infants are born underweight, mentally retarded, and with behavioral, facial, limb, heart, and nervous system defects. Women who smoke run a statistically higher risk of miscarrying. If they don't miscarry, chances are good their babies will be born smaller than average and will continue to be smaller than children of nonsmoking mothers even well into childhood. More recently, some studies have indicated that the caffeine in a daily cup of coffee might also increase the chances for abnormal fetal development.

Pregnant women are also well advised to avoid exposure to x-ray examinations. Early in pregnancy, x-rays can increase the risk of miscarriage, and also possibly cause an increase in fetal malformations. Abdominal x-ray examinations of pregnant women late in pregnancy to determine the size and position of the fetus increases that unborn child's risk for developing leukemia. According to the FDA's Bureau of Radiological Health, a child exposed to x-radiation before birth has a risk of about one in one thousand for developing leukemia as a result.

Although most drugs can and should be avoided by pregnant women without question, pregnant women who need medical treatment are still left with a dreadful dilemma—to take the suggested treatment and risk harming the unborn child or refuse the drug and risk perhaps losing the unborn child. Before making any decision regarding medical treatment during pregnancy, the woman should get from her doctor all the information he or she has about the risks of the treatment versus the benefits. Sometimes, simply listing these side by side can make the decision to accept or refuse treatment a foregone conclusion. If there is no clear choice, then a woman should not hesitate to seek a second opinion, preferably from an obstetrician who specializes in high-risk pregnancies. Most state medical societies can help consumers find such a specialist. The pregnant woman with a true medical emergency has no choice but to accept necessary life- or health-saving measures. Fortunately, such dire situations are the exception rather than the rule.

But for the vast majority of pregnant women, drugs are the enemy. In the nineteenth century, Sir William Osler, a distinguished physician and philosopher, said, "The desire to take medicine is perhaps the greatest feature which distinguishes man from the animals." During pregnancy, at least, women would do well to take a lesson from the animal kingdom.

# 10 · What Every Consumer Should Know To Get Safer and Better Health Care

*"Truth in all its kinds is most difficult to win; and truth in medicine is the most difficult of all."*

Peter Mere Latham (1789–1875)

The ultimate question that must be asked of any mistake is, "What has it taught us?" Can we learn from the DES experience to be less vulnerable to medical mistakes? The answer is a resounding "Yes!"

People who are uninitiated in science and medicine can still become more effective health care consumers by understanding their weaknesses, their rights, their resources, and their responsibilities as patients.

Illness, or the threat of illness, places a unique burden upon the consumer. In an otherwise consumer-oriented society, the health care establishment alone—and in particular, the physician—remains sacrosanct. Illness is the consumers' Achilles' heel rendering them vulnerable emotionally and intellectually as well as physically. But this helplessness, as intrinsic as it may seem to the situation, need not and should not be a necessary part of the doctor-patient relationship.

## • DISPELLING THE MYTHS

The first step toward a more effective partnership between the health care consumer (the patient) and the health care provider (the physician) is to dispel the myths that complicate and distort this relationship. At least two myths are pervasive and ultimately damage the quality of medical care.

*Myth #1: The physician is a superior being.* Underlying the relationship between most doctors and most patients is an unwritten, but firmly entrenched, caste system. The myth involves a general assumption on the part of both doctor and patient that the doctor is intrinsically superior to the patient.

In a way, this is true. The patient, after all, goes to the doctor for the special knowledge and skills that the doctor possesses and that the patient does not. So, within the context of the hospital or the doctor's office or the clinic or the sickbed, the doctor is indeed preeminent—preeminent in his or her special environment, much as a plumber is preeminent when a pipe is leaking, or a lawyer is preeminent in the courtroom, or a mechanic is preeminent when a car breaks down. Each is a specialist with skills to alleviate special problems. However, beyond the context of their skills, most "specialists" are generally regarded as ordinary people.

But not so with the physician. Doctors generate a mystique that often gets them better seats in theaters, better suites in hotels, better tables at restaurants, even though none of these activities has anything to do with medicine. This mystique is merely symptomatic of myth #1, which derives in part from the fact that the physician bares and probes people's bodies and not merely their possessions. Under these circumstances, it is only human to seek to justify this nakedness and vulnerability by imputing to the physician a superiority that is absolute, similar to the feeling most children have for their parents.

Second, the mystique springs from an ancient association between health care and the supernatural. Shamans, witch doctors, and faith healers have all commanded considerable respect for their alleged powers to heal, whether by divine grace or by supernatural powers.

In an article titled "God and the Doctor," published in the

*New England Journal of Medicine,* Dr. Humphrey Osmond examined the often extraordinary authority vested in physicians. One of the elements of this authority, explained Dr. Osmond, is "charismatic," authority that people generally accept as being derived from a kind of "God-given grace." This element of a physician's authority, according to Osmond, springs from the physician's "priestly role" in mediating and/or controlling the unknowns of illness, as well as the possibility of death.

This leaves patients feeling pretty helpless with little else to do but try to curry favor! The stage is further set for myth #1 in the examining room where the physician is the high priest and the patient the humble supplicant. The physician, fully clothed and coated in dazzling white, is suitably depersonalized behind the title of "Doctor" while the patient, "Jim" or "Jane," lies supine and shivering inside a gaping hospital "johnnie"!

Understanding these emotional aspects of the doctor-patient relationship can help the health care consumer to become a more effective patient.

*Myth #2: Women are neurotics and hypochondriacs.* For all the gains made in equal rights in the past two decades, sexism is alive and kicking in the hearts of too many doctors everywhere. And it is affecting the quality of health care that women receive.

Eleanor Smeal, president of the National Organization of Women (NOW), told a U.S. Senate Subcommittee on Health and Scientific Research that "sex-stereotyped thinking about women accounts for many of the scandals in abuse of health care delivery."

She cited Caesarean sections, hysterectomies, and radical mastectomies as three examples of procedures unique to women that have been performed excessively and unnecessarily. In 1968, only 5 percent of all deliveries were by Caesarean section; by 1976, this percentage had risen to 11.6 percent. This increase, said Ms. Smeal, was not accompanied by a corresponding decrease in infant mortality.

As for hysterectomies, the necessity for many of them was questioned as long ago as 1946. A paper published in the *American Journal of Obstetrics and Gynecology* in that year decried the high number of "unjustified" hysterectomies. The paper, titled "Hysterectomy: Therapeutic Necessity or Surgical Racket?" reported the results of a study of hysterectomies performed at 10 different hospitals during the first four months of 1945. The reviewers learned that 246 such operations were performed, and concluded that at least half of these were "unjustified." Now, more than 35 years later, published reports are still appearing that indicate that unnecessary hysterectomies continue to be performed regularly.

Although the benefits of radical mastectomy over less disfiguring surgery have been roundly challenged for at least a decade, one-fourth of all mastectomies performed in this country are still radical ones. (*See* chapter 6.)

In 1979, three California medical researchers decided to formally study charges of "alleged sexism" in the medical profession. They studied health records of 52 married couples, all of whom received medical care from the same group practice of nine male physicians. In evaluating five common complaints—back pain, headache, dizziness, chest pain, and fatigue—the three researchers found that the physicians' examinations were significantly more extensive for their men patients than for their women patients. The three concluded that their study supported popular claims that male physicians tend to take illness more seriously in men than in women.

"In doing so," they wrote in *JAMA*, "the doctors might be responding to current stereotypes that regard the male as typically stoical and the female as typically hypochondriacal."

Dispelling the myth of the neurotic female patient will take the cooperation and concerted efforts of women's groups, government officials, and sensitive physicians. For the individual woman faced with a chauvinistic male doctor, her only effective alternative in terms of getting quality health care may be to change physicians.

# • LEARNING YOUR RIGHTS AS A PATIENT

A right is something to which you are entitled either by law or by commonly accepted ethical standards. Knowing your medical rights can make the difference between effective and fairly priced medical treatment or prolonged illness and unfair expense.

Many health care consumers are not aware that they have certain rights as patients. The following Patient's Bill of Rights was formulated by the American Hospital Association in consultation with its Regional Advisory Board and consumer representatives. It was first published in January 1973.

### The AHA Patient Bill of Rights

1. The patient has the right to considerate and respectful care.

2. The patient has the right to obtain from his physician complete current information concerning his diagnosis, treatment, and prognosis in terms the patient can reasonably be expected to understand.

3. The patient has the right to receive from his physician information necessary to give informed consent prior to the start of any procedure or treatment.

4. The patient has the right to refuse treatment to the extent permitted by law, and to be informed of the medical consequences of his action. [The patient might *not* have the right to refuse treatment if, for example, he poses a health danger to others; or, a parent might not have the right to refuse medical treatment on behalf of a child.]

5. The patient has the right to every consideration of his privacy concerning his own medical care program.

6. The patient has the right to expect that all communications and records pertaining to his care should be treated as confidential.

7. The patient has the right to expect that within its capacity, a hospital must make reasonable response to the request of a patient for services.

8. The patient has the right to obtain information as to

any relationship of his hospital to other health care and educational institutions insofar as his care is concerned.

9. The patient has the right to be advised if the hospital proposes to engage in or perform human experimentation affecting his care or treatment.

10. The patient has the right to expect reasonable continuity of care.

11. The patient has the right to examine and receive an explanation of his bill regardless of source of payment.

12. The patient has the right to know what hospital rules and regulations apply to his conduct as a patient.

If a patient believes that his or her rights have been violated, he should enlist the help of a doctor or nurse he can trust. Or, if in a hospital, ask to speak with the hospital's patient representative. Many larger hospitals employ special people to act as patient ombudsmen, and can help the patient redress grievances.

*Patient arbitration agreements.* The Coalition for the Medical Rights of Women of San Francisco warns patients about signing agreements that abrogate their legal rights in cases of medical negligence or malpractice. The coalition warns that some doctors and some medical groups require patients to sign arbitration agreements which, in effect, remove the right of the patient to sue the doctor in a court of law. If the patient has a grievance, the case is then tried privately, before a panel of privately chosen arbitrators. Consumers should carefully weigh the pros and cons of such agreements *before* signing.

*Living wills.* A living will is a document not unlike a property will. Only the living will contains instructions for how a person would like him- or herself cared for in case he becomes incapacitated. The living will is signed in the presence of witnesses and should be notarized. Many people began to feel the need for such documents as medical care and technology grew more sophisticated, and the lives of terminally ill or incapacitated persons were prolonged—often with great suffering—solely by virtue of advanced technologies and medical treatments.

Often, these patients are so ill they are unable to speak for themselves. Many people who anticipate the possibility of such an illness prepare a living will, which stipulates the kind and degree of medical treatment they wish to receive if they should become seriously ill; or, the will may contain instruction that *no* treatment be given to prolong life and suffering when there is no hope of recovery.

*Your access rights to your medical records.* There has been a traditional aversion on the part of the medical profession to allow patients access to their own medical records. For some patients, such access is imperative. DES mothers and daughters, for example, need to be able to ascertain if, when, and for how long they were exposed to DES.

Policy regarding patient access to medical records varies widely, from state to state as well as from clinic to clinic. However, it is generally recognized, says Meryl Bloomrosen, a medical records specialist, that while the physician owns the actual record, the patient owns the information contained in the records.

Patients who are denied access to their medical records can turn to several places for help. The first is a state Department of Health. Often, this department can clarify for the patient whether or not a state statute specifically accords patients the right of access. If so, then a health department official can call the clinic on behalf of the patient.

Two potentially helpful organizations recommended by Ms. Bloomrosen are the American Medical Record Association, 875 North Michigan Avenue, Chicago, Ill. 60611 and the Public Citizen's Health Research Group, 2000 P Street, N.W., Washington D.C. 20036.

## • KNOWING YOUR RESOURCES

The past decade has seen an explosion of health care information written for the consumer on every conceivable health subject from holistic medicine to do-it-yourself gynecological examinations. However helpful these may be, the average health care consumer will still rely upon his or her physician for health care needs. So, ultimately the most valuable books for many people will be those that help them to work more effectively within the general framework of the doctor-patient relationship.

The following books are described as examples of their kind. There are many other fine books as well on the shelves of bookstores and libraries, which the reader is encouraged to use.

Among the most potentially helpful books are those that explain and describe drugs. Some of these books are written for use by the medical profession, and a few are written for the lay public. Whichever you choose, drug information books can prove invaluable.

*The Physician's Desk Reference (PDR)*, published annually by Medical Economics Company, Oradell, N.J., is considered an indispensable aid by practicing physicians. It contains information about every drug—both prescription and over-the-counter—that is approved for sale in this country. Although the information on each drug is supplied by the drug companies themselves, the manufacturers are required by law to publish *all* information—including adverse side effects—as well as beneficial effects. The *PDR* is cross-indexed by brand name, by generic drug name, and by type of drug (such as hormones, vitamins, antibiotics, and so on).

Although the language is technical, most of the content of the *PDR* can be unraveled by a medical dictionary. The *PDR* should be available in most libraries.

There are, as well, drug reference books written specifically for a nonscientific readership which consumers may also find helpful.

*The Best Doctors in the U.S.*, by John Pekkanen (Seaview Books, 1979), seemed destined to be buried under an avalanche of lawsuits issued by howling mobs of irate physicians. This most dire of consequences has not happened and this listing (real names and addresses of physicians all over the country) is a bona fide catalog of top-notch doctors. The editor of this ambitious book compiled his list from hundreds of questionnaires sent out to physicians in all parts of the country, and in every medical specialty. The physicians were asked to name the doctors *they* would go to if they developed various medical problems. (The consumer can apply this same technique on a small scale when searching for a new doctor.)

Each of the following books offers valuable advice to the consumer. These books are only a sampling of the wealth of information and good advice readily available to everyone.

*Talk Back To Your Doctor: How to Demand (& Recognize) High Quality Health Care,* by Arthur Levin, M.D. (Doubleday, New York), delivers exactly what the title promises! In clearly witten, straightforward lay language, the author, a Harvard Medical School graduate, tells his readers exactly *how* to talk with physicians to demystify health care and make it work more effectively for them.

*Straight Talk About Your Health Care: How to Understand and Use the World of Modern Medicine,* by Mack Lipkin, M.D. (Harper & Row, New York, 1977), is also written in easy to understand language. It contains information about the process of diagnosing an illness, insights into how the physician arrives at a diagnosis, lay explanations of different groups of drugs, such as antibiotics, hormones, and tranquilizers, as well as criteria for choosing a physician.

*The People's Hospital Book: How to Increase Your Comfort and Safety, Deal with Nurses and Doctors, and Obtain the Best Total Care,* by Ronald Gots, M.D., Ph.D., and Arthur Kaufman, M.D. (Crown, New York, 1978). This book deals exclusively with hospital care. It tells the consumer how to choose a hospital, how to judge the competence of the surgeon, how to get along with the nursing staff, all about hospital procedures and equipment, a guide to special care units, and how to prepare a child for hospitalization.

Remember, these brief book reviews are only examples of many excellent books which are readily available.

*Self-help groups.* Health care consumers may also avail themselves of any one or more of a growing number of groups, called self-help groups, which are generally composed of consumers and are devoted solely to a specific health problem. These groups have usually been started by lay persons who have been personally affected by a particular medical problem, which may range from the commonplace such as heart disease to the more exotic such as retinitis pigmentosa.

Although these groups vary in the number of members, their budgets, or their internal structures, they all share the common purpose of helping people affected by a special problem.

DES Action, Inc., is a national consumer organization concerned with every aspect of DES exposure. It offers information, education, and support for DES-exposed individuals. It also monitors and lobbies for state and federal legislation concerning DES, and provides information to attorneys and litigants. The group publishes a quarterly newsletter as well as a number of brochures designed to give an overview of various DES-associated problems. The nominal annual membership of $15 (as of 1981) entitles members to these publications which contain a wealth of relevant information and advice.

The group has an East Coast office in New York and a West Coast office in San Francisco, as well as local chapters throughout the country. It is administered by an executive director and is governed by a board of directors. Consultants to the organization include nationally prominent medical, legal, and lay experts.

For more information, contact either one of the national offices or a local chapter. (*See* appendix for addresses.)

### • *YOUR RESPONSIBILITIES AS A PATIENT*

No litany of rights and resources—however complete—can fully insure good health care without a parallel exercise of patient responsibilities.

To be an effective consumer of health care services, the adult patient must make his or her association with the physician an active partnership. He or she must ask questions (even if the questions seem foolish), use consumer resources, and not hesitate to get second or even third medical opinions when there is any doubt.

While there will always be some physicians who will interpret an activist patient as a threat to his authority and an insult to his expertise, remember there will also be physicians who will welcome the patient's active and sincere participation in health care delivery.

Can we avoid the mistakes of the past? Can we be more astute and effective health care consumers? We can if we are prepared to act in our own behalves, if we are prepared to assume a more active role in our own health care, and if we remember that there are no easy answers and that Panacea is just a name from Greek mythology.

Nothing more.

# Bibliography

## CHAPTER 2

1 Asimov, Isaac: *The Intelligent Man's Guide to Science, Vol. 2, The Biological Sciences.* Basic Books, Inc., New York, 1960.

2 Bethune, John E: *The Adrenal Cortex.* A Scope Monograph, edited by Baird A. Thomas, The Upjohn Co., Kalamazoo, 1974.

3 Burdick HO; Vedder, Helen: The effect of stilbestrol in early pregnancy. *Endocrinology,* Vol. 28: p. 629, 1941.

4 Connally HF Jr; Dann DI; Reese JM; et al: A clinical study of the effects of diethylstilbestrol on puerperal women. *American Journal of Obstetrics and Gynecology,* Vol. 40: p. 445, 1940.

5 Corea, Gena: *The Hidden Malpractice (How American Medicine Treats Women as Patients and Professionals).* William Morrow and Company, Inc., New York, 1977.

6 DeCoursey, Russell Myles: *The Human Organism,* Chapter 20, "The Endocrine System," McGraw Hill Book Company, Inc., New York, 1961.

7 Dieckmann WJ; Davis ME; Rynkiewicz LM; Pottinger RE: Does the administration of diethylstilbestrol during pregnancy have therapeutic value? *American Journal of Obstetrics and Gynecology,* Vol. 66 (no. 5): p. 1062, Nov. 1953.

8 Dodds EC: Biologic effects of the synthetic oestrogenic substance 4:4'-dihydroxy-alph: beta-diethylstilbene, *Lancet,* p. 1389, June 18, 1938.

9 Ferguson JH: Effects of stilbestrol on pregnancy compared to the effect of a placebo. *American Journal of Obstetrics and Gynecology,* Vol. 65: p. 592, 1953.

10 Guyton, Arthur C: *Textbook of Medical Physiology,* Part X, "Endocrinology," W. B. Saunders Company, Philadelphia, 1956.

11 Haire, Doris: *The Cultural Warping of Childbirth.* A special issue. International Childbirth Education Association, 1972.

12 Hamblen EC: Some contributions of endocrinology to obstetrics and gynecology. *American Journal of Obstetrics and Gynecology,* Vol. 51 (no. 6): p. 796, June 1946.

13 Heinonen OP: Diethylstilbestrol in pregnancy: frequency of exposure and usage patterns. *Cancer,* Vol. 31 (no. 3): p. 573, March 1973.

14 *IARC Monographs on the Evaluation of the Carcinogenic Risk of Chemicals to Man,* Vol. 6, "The Sex Hormones," section on Diethylstilbestrol. Published by the International Agency for Research on Cancer (a working agency of the World Health Organization), Lyons, France, 1974.

15 Lacassagne A: Apparition d'adenocarcinomes mammaires chez des souris mâles traitées par une substance oestrogène synthetique. *Comptes Rendus Biol.* (Paris), Vol. 129: p. 641, 1938.

16 Medical News column: Painless thyroiditis is often missed as postpartum depression cause. *JAMA,* Vol. 237 (no. 11): p. 1065, March 14, 1977.

17 Muckle CW: The suppression of lactation by stilbestrol. *American Journal of Obstetrics and Gynecology,* Vol. 40: p. 133, 1940.

18 Noller KL; Fish CR: Diethylstilbestrol usage: its interesting past, important present, and questionable future. *Medical Clinics of North America,* Vol. 58 (no. 40): p. 793, July 1974.

19 Payne FL; Muckle CW: Stilbestrol in the treatment of menopausal symptoms. *American Journal of Obstetrics and Gynecology,* Vol. 40: p. 135, 1940.

20 Reddoch JW; Wiener WB: Stilbestrol in the termination of pregnancy. *American Journal of Obstetrics and Gynecology,* Vol. 45 (no. 2): p. 343, February 1943.

21 Russ JS; Collins CG: The treatment of prepubertal vulvovaginitis with a new synthetic estrogen. *JAMA,* Vol. 114: p. 2446, 1940.

22 Seaman, Barbara and Seaman, Gideon: *Women and the Crisis in Sex Hormones.* Rawson Associates Publishers, Inc., New York, 1977.

23 Selye H: On the toxicity of oestrogens with special reference to diethylstilbestrol. *Canadian Medical Association Journal,* Vol. 41: p. 48, 1939.

24 Shimkin MB; Grady HL: Mammary carcinomas in mice following oral administration of stilbestrol. *Proceedings of the Society for Experimental Biology and Medicine,* Vol. 45: p. 246, 1940.

25 Smith GVS; Smith OW: Observations concerning the metabolism of estrogens in women. *American Journal of Obstetrics and Gynecology,* Vol. 36 (no. 5): p. 769, November 1938.

26 Smith GVS; Smith OW: Prophylactic hormone therapy: relation to complications of pregnancy. *Obstetrics and Gynecology,* Vol. 4 (no. 2): p. 129, August 1954.

27 Smith OW; Smith GVS; Hurwitz D: Increased excretion of pregnanediol in pregnancy from diethylstilbestrol with special reference to the preven-

tion of late pregnancy accidents. *American Journal of Obstetrics and Gynecology,* Vol. 51 (no. 3): p. 411, March 1946.

28 Smith OW: Diethylstilbestrol in the prevention and treatment of complications of pregnancy. *American Journal of Obstetrics and Gynecology,* Vol. 56 (no. 5): p. 821, November 1948.

## CHAPTER 3

1 Antonioli DA; Burke L; Friedman EA: Natural history of diethylstilbestrol-associated genital tract lesions; cervical ectopy and cervicovaginal hood. *American Journal of Obstetrics and Gynecology,* Vol. 137: p. 847, August 1, 1980.

2 Associated Press: Scientist says DES may start cancer. *The Capital Times* (Madison, Wisconsin), May 11, 1979.

3 Burke L; Antonioli DA; Rosen S: Vaginal and cervical cell dysplasia in women exposed to diethylstilbestrol in utero. *American Journal of Obstetrics and Gynecology,* Vol. 38: p. 426, 1976.

4 *Clinical Oncology for Medical Students and Physicians,* "Carcinoma of the Vagina," (p. 248), published by the University of Rochester School of Medicine and Dentistry, Rochester, 1974.

5 Fetherston WC: Squamous neoplasia of vaginal related to DES syndrome. *American Journal of Obstetrics and Gynecology,* p. 176, May 15, 1975.

6 Forsberg JG: Late effects in the vaginal and cervical epithelia after injections of diethylstilbestrol into neonatal mice. *American Journal of Obstetrics and Gynecology,* pp. 101–104, January 1, 1975.

7 Greenwald P; Barlow JJ; Nasca PC; Burnett WS: Vaginal cancer after maternal treatment with synthetic estrogens. *New England Journal of Medicine,* Vol. 285 (no. 7): p. 390, August 12, 1971.

8 Herbst AL; Ulfelder H; Poskanzer DC: Adenocarcinoma of the vagina. Association of maternal stilbestrol therapy with tumor appearance in young women. *New England Journal of Medicine,* Vol. 284 (no. 16): pp. 878–881, April 22, 1971.

9 Herbst AL; Cole P: Epidemiologic and clinical aspects of clear cell adenocarcinoma in young women. Proceedings of the Symposium on DES, May 6, 1977, sponsored by the American College of Obstetricians and Gynecologists.

10 Herbst AL: *1979–1980 Newsletter.* Published by the Registry for Research on Hormonal Transplacental Carcinogenesis, Chicago.

11 Herbst AL; Cole PL; Colton T; Robboy SJ; Scully RE: Age-incidence and risk of diethylstilbestrol-related clear cell adenocarcinoma of the vagina and cervix. *American Journal of Obstetrics and Gynecology*, Vol. 128 (no. 1): pp. 43–50, May 1, 1977.

12 Herbst AL; Cole PL; Norusis MJ; Welch WR; Scully RE: Epidemiologic aspects and factors related to survival in 384 Registry cases of clear cell adenocarcinoma of the vagina and cervix. *American Journal of Obstetrics and Gynecology*, Vol. 135 (no. 7): p. 876, December 1, 1979.

13 Herbst AL; Norusis MJ; Rosenow PH; Welch WR; Scully RE: An analysis of 346 cases of clear cell adenocarcinoma of the vagina and cervix with emphasis on recurrence and survival. *Gynecologic Oncology*, Vol. 7: pp. 111–122, 1979.

14 Donahue, Dorothy: DES: a case study. *Cancer Nursing*, p. 207, June 1978.

15 Herbst AL; Scully RE; Robboy SJ; Welch WR: Complications of prenatal therapy with diethylstilbestrol. *Pediatrics* (supplement), Vol. 62 (no. 6): part 2: p. 1151, December 1978.

16 Hillemanns HG; Bauknecht T; Simmer H: The stilbestrol-adenosis-carcinoma syndrome. *Obstetrical and Gynecological Survey*, Vol. 34 (no. 11): p. 814, 1979.

17 Lanier AP; Noller KL; Decker DG; Elveback LR; Kurland LT: Cancer and stilbestrol—a follow-up of 1,719 persons exposed to estrogens in utero and born 1943–1959. *Mayo Clinic Proceedings*, Vol. 48: p. 793, November 1973.

18 Medical News: Risk of cancer, dysplasia for DES daughters found "very low." *JAMA*, April 13, 1979.

19 Nordqvist SRB; Fidler WJ Jr; Woodruff JM; Lewis JL: Clear cell adenocarcinoma of the cervix and vagina. A clinico-pathologic study of 21 cases with and without a history of maternal ingestion of estrogens. *Cancer*, Vol. 37: pp. 858–871, 1979.

20 Professional and Public Relations Committee of the DESAD Project of the National Cancer Institute and the Office of Cancer Communications NCI. Questions and Answers About DES Exposure Before Birth. U.S. Dept. of Health, Education, and Welfare Publication No. (NIH) 76-1118.

21 Richart RM; Fu YS; Reagan JW; Barron BA: The problem of squamous neoplasia in female DES progeny. Chapter 6 of *Proceedings of "Symposium on DES," 1977*, published by the American College of Obstetricians and Gynecologists, February 1978.

22 Sandberg EC; Christian JC: Diethylstilbestrol-exposed monozygotic

twins discordant for cervicovaginal clear cell adenocarcinoma. *American Journal of Obstetrics and Gynecology,* Vol. 137: p. 220, May 15, 1980.

23 Scully R; Robboy SJ; Welch WR: Pathology and pathogenesis of diethylstilbestrol-related disorders of the female genital tract. Chapter 2 of *Proceedings of "Symposium on DES," 1977.* Edited by Dr. Arthur L. Herbst, published by the American College of Obstetricians and Gynecologists, February 1978.

24 Stafl A: Squamous neoplasia in DES-exposed women. *Obstetrical and Gynecological Survey.* Vol. 34 (no. 11): p. 847, 1979.

25 Stafl A; Mattingly RF; Foley DV; Fetherston WC: Clinical diagnosis of vaginal adenosis. *Obstetrics and Gynecology,* Vol. 43 (no. 1): p. 118, January 1974.

26 Stafl A; Mattingly RF: Vaginal adenosis; a precancerous lesion? *American Journal of Obstetrics and Gynecology,* Vol. 120 (no. 5): pp. 666–673, November 1, 1974.

27 Ulfelder H: The stilbestrol-adenosis-carcinoma syndrome. *Cancer,* Vol. 38: p. 426, 1976.

In addition to the above references, parts of chapter 3 are based on an interview with Adolf Stafl, M.D., on August 11, 1980.

## CHAPTER 4

1 Anderson B; Watring WG; Edinger DD; Small EC; Netland AT; Saffaii H: Development of DES-associated clear-cell carcinoma; the importance of regular screening. *Obstetrics and Gynecology,* Vol. 53 (no. 3): pp. 293–299, March 1979.

2 Barbar HRK: DES-exposed offspring: how you can help. (Editorial) *The Female Patient,* p. 9, August 1977.

3 Barnes AB: Menstrual history of young women exposed in utero to diethylstilbestrol. *Fertility and Sterility,* Vol. 32 (no. 2): p. 148, August 1979.

4 Barnes AB; Colton T; Gundersen J; Noller KL; Tilley BC; Strama T; Townsend DE; Hatab P; O'Brien PC: Fertility and outcome of pregnancy in women exposed in utero to diethylstilbestrol. *New England Journal of Medicine,* Vol. 302 (no. 11): p. 609, March 13, 1980.

5 Berger MJ; Goldstein DP: Impaired reproductive performance in DES-exposed women. *Obstetrics and Gynecology,* Vol. 55 (no. 1): p. 25, January 1980.

6 Burghardt E; Holzer E: Treatment of carcinoma in situ; evaluation of 1609 cases. *Obstetrics and Gynecology,* Vol. 55 (no. 5): pp. 539–545, May 1980.

7 Burke L; Apfel RJ; Fisher S; Shaw J: Observations on the psychological impact of diethylstilbestrol exposure and suggestions on management. *The Journal of Reproductive Medicine,* Vol. 24 (no. 3): p. 99, March 1980.

8 Burke L; Antonioli D; Friedman EA: Evolution of diethylstilbestrol-associated genital tract lesions. *Obstetrics and Gynecology,* Vol. 57 (no. 1): pp. 79–84, January 1981.

9 Chan CR; Detmer D: Proper management of hepatic adenomas associated with oral contraceptives. *Surgery, Gynecology & Obstetrics,* Vol. 44: p. 703, 1977.

10 Charles EH; Savage EW: Cryosurgical treatment of cervical intraepithelial neoplasia. *Obstetrical and Gynecological Survey,* Vol. 35 (no. 9): pp. 539–547, 1980.

11 Corsello, Serafina: Speech on the Emotional Trauma of DES Exposure in Teen-Age Girls. Delivered to the Physician-Professional Health Education Seminar sponsored by the California Board of Health and the American Cancer Society, San Francisco, June 3, 1977.

12 Cousins L; Karp W; Lacey C; Lucas WE: Reproductive outcome of women exposed to diethylstilbestrol in utero. *Obstetrics and Gynecology,* Vol. 56 (no. 1): p. 70, July 1980.

13 DES Task Force Summary Report, Part II—DES Daughters, September 21, 1978.

14 Ehrhardt Anke A: Behavioral effects of estrogen in the human female. *Pediatrics,* Vol. 62 (no. 6): p. 1166, December 1978.

15 Fishbane, Fran: Emotional Problems in the DES Exposed. (Speech—text provided by DES Action).

16 Fowler WC; Edelman DA: In utero exposure to DES. Evaluation and follow-up of 199 women. *Obstetrics and Gynecology.* Vol. 51 (no. 4): pp. 459–463, April 1978.

17 Goldstein DP: Incompetent cervix in offspring exposed to diethylstilbestrol in utero. *Obstetrics and Gynecology,* Vol. 52 (no. 1): p. 73, July 1978.

18 Haney AF; Hammond CB; Soules MR; Creasman WT: Diethylstilbestrol-induced upper genital tract abnormalities. *Fertility and Sterility,* Vol. 31 (no. 2): p. 142, February 1979.

19 Hart WR; Townsend DE; Aldrich JO; Henderson BE; Roy M; Benton B: Histopathologic spectrum of vaginal adenosis and related changes in stilbestrol-exposed females. *Cancer,* Vol. 37: p. 763, February 1976.

20 Herbst AL; Scully RE; Robboy SJ; Welch WR: Complications of prenatal therapy with diethylstilbestrol. *Pediatrics* (supplement), Vol. 62 (no. 6): part 2: p. 1151, December 1978.

21 Herbst AL; Hubby MM; Blough RR; Azizi F: A comparison of pregnancy experience in DES-exposed and DES-unexposed daughters. *The Journal of Reproductive Medicine*, Vol. 124 (no. 2): p. 62, February 1980.

22 Hulka BS; Fowler WC; Kaufman DG; et al: Estrogen and endometrial cancer: cases and two control groups from North Carolina. *American Journal of Obstetrics and Gynecology*, Vol. 137: p. 92, May 1, 1980.

23 Kaufman RH; Adam E; Grey MP; Gerthoffer E: Urinary tract changes associated with exposure in utero to diethylstilbestrol. *Obstetrics and Gynecology*, Vol. 56 (no. 3): p. 330, September 1980.

24 Kaufman RH; Binder GL; Gray PM; Adam E: Upper genital tract changes associated with exposure in utero to diethylstilbestrol. *American Journal of Obstetrics and Gynecology*, Vol. 128: p. 51, May 1, 1977.

25 Koss, Leopold: Dysplasia. A real concept or a misnomer? *Obstetrics and Gynecology*, Vol. 51 (no. 3): pp. 374–379, March 1978.

26 Krumholz BA: The $CO_2$ Laser. DES Action *Voice*, Vol. 1 (no. 3): p. 3, Summer 1979.

27 Magrina JF; Masterson BJ: Vaginal reconstruction in gynecological oncology; A review of techniques. *Obstetrical and Gynecological Survey*, Vol. 36 (no. 1): pp. 1–10, January 1981.

28 Meyer-Bahlburg HFL: Behavioral effects of estrogen treatments in human males. *Pediatrics* (supplement), Vol. 62 (no. 6): part 2: p. 1171, December 1978.

29 Mylotte MJ; Allen JM; Jordan JA: Regeneration of cervical epithelium following laser destruction of intraepithelial neoplasia. *Obstetrical and Gynecological Survey*, Vol. 34 (no. 11): pp. 859–860, November 1979.

30 Neuberger J; Protmann B; Nunnerley HB; et al: Oral contraceptive-associated liver tumors: Occurrence of malignancy and difficulties in diagnosis. *Lancet*, Vol. 1: p. 273, 1980.

31 Nunley WC; Kitchin JD: Successful management of incompetent cervix in a primigravida exposed to diethylstilbestrol in utero. *Fertility and Sterility*, Vol. 31 (no. 2): p. 217, February 1979.

32 O'Brien PC; Noller KL; Robboy SJ; Barnes AB; Kaufman RH; Tilley BC; Townsend DE: Vaginal epithelial changes in young women enrolled in the

National Cooperative Diethylstilbestrol Adenosis (DESAD) Project. *Obstetrics and Gynecology,* Vol. 53 (no. 3): p. 300, March 1979.

33 Pillsbury SG Jr: Reproductive significance of changes in the endometrial cavity associated with exposure in utero to diethylstilbestrol. *American Journal of Obstetrics and Gynecology,* Vol. 137 (no. 2): p. 178, May 15, 1980.

34 Richart RM; Townsend DE; Crisp W; et al: An analysis of "long-term" follow-up results in patients with cervical intraepithelial neoplasia treated by cryotherapy. *American Journal of Obstetrics and Gynecology,* Vol. 137: pp. 823–826, 1980.

35 Rosenfeld DL; Bronson RA: Reproductive problems in the DES-exposed female. *Obstetrics and Gynecology,* Vol. 55 (no. 4): p. 453, April 1980.

36 Sandberg EC: Benign cervical and vaginal changes associated with exposure to stilbestrol in utero. *American Journal of Obstetrics and Gynecology,* Vol. 125 (no. 6): p. 778, July 15, 1976.

37 Sandberg EC; Hebard JC: Examination of young women exposed to stilbestrol in utero. *American Journal of Obstetrics and Gynecology,* Vol. 128: p. 364, 1977.

38 Schmidt G; Fowler WC; Talbert LM; Edelman DA: Reproductive history of women exposed to diethylstilbestrol in utero. *Fertility and Sterility,* Vol. 33: p. 21, January 1980.

39 Schmidt G; Fowler WC Jr: Cervical stenosis following minor gynecologic procedures on DES-exposed women. *Obstetrics and Gynecology,* Vol. 56 (no. 3): pp. 333–335, September 1980.

40 Schwartz RW; Stewart N: Psychological effects of diethylstilbestrol exposure. *JAMA,* Vol. 237 (no. 3): p. 252, January 17, 1977.

41 Siegler AM; Wang CF; Friberg J: Fertility of the diethylstilbestrol-exposed offspring. *Fertility and Sterility,* Vol. 31 (no. 6): p. 601, June 1979.

42 Stafl A; Wilkinson EJ; Mattingly RF: Laser treatment of cervical and vaginal neoplasia. *American Journal of Obstetrics and Gynecology,* Vol. 128: p. 128, 1977.

43 Townsend DE: Techniques of examination and screening of the DES-exposed female. Chapter 3 of *Intrauterine Exposure to Diethylstilbestrol in the Human. Proceedings of "Symposium on DES," 1977.* Edited by Dr. Arthur L. Herbst; the American College of Obstetricians and Gynecologists, Chicago, February 1978.

44 Ulfelder H: The current status of stilbestrol disorders. *Surgical Rounds,* pp. 50–53, January 1979.

45 Weber T; Obel E: Pregnancy complications following conization of the uterine cervix. *Obstetrical and Gynecological Survey*, Vol. 35 (no. 5): pp. 287–289, May 1980.

46 Weiss NS; Sayvetz TA: Incidence of endometrial cancer in relation to the use of oral contraceptives. *The New England Journal of Medicine*, Vol. 302 (no. 10): p. 551, March 6, 1980.

47 Wilson WE; Agrawal AK: Brain regional levels of neurotransmitter amines as neurochemical correlates of sex-specific ontongenesis in the rat. *Developmental Neuroscience*, Vol. 2 (no. 4): pp. 195–200, 1979.

In addition to the above references, material for this chapter was taken from personal interviews with Hannah Cook-Wallace and Andrea Goldstein.

## CHAPTER 5

1 Abrams HJ: Genital and semen abnormalities in adolescent males exposed to DES. *JCAM*, p. 44, July 1980.

2 Anderson T: Testicular germ-cell neoplasms: recent advances in diagnosis and therapy. *Annals of Internal Medicine*, Vol. 50: p. 373, 1979.

3 Bibbo M; Al-Naquub M; Baccarini I; Gill W; Newton M; Sleeper KM; Sonek M; Wied GL: Follow-up study of male and female offspring of DES-treated mothers; a preliminary report. *Journal of Reproductive Medicine*, Vol. 15 (no. 1): p. 29, July 1975.

4 Bibbo M; Gill WB; Azizi F; Blough R; Fang VS; Rosenfield RL; Schumacker GB; Sleeper K; Sonek MG; Wied GL: Follow-up study of male and female offspring of DES-exposed mothers. *Obstetrics and Gynecology*, Vol. 49 (no. 1): p. 1, January 1977.

5 Cosgrove MD; Benton B; Henderson BE: Male genitourinary abnormalities and maternal diethylstilbestrol. *The Journal of Urology*, Vol. 117: pp. 220–222, 1977.

6 D'Orner G; Stahl F; Rohde W; Schnorr D: An apparently direct inhibitory effect of oestrogen on the human testis. *Endokrinologie*, Vol. 66 (no. 2): pp. 221–224, 1975.

7 Driscoll SG; Taylor SH: Effects of prenatal maternal estrogen on the male urogenital system. *Obstetrics and Gynecology*, Vol. 56 (no. 5): pp. 47–50, November 1980.

8 Einhorn LH; Donohue JP: Combination chemotherapy in disseminated testicular cancer; the Indiana University experience. *Seminars in Oncology,* Vol. 6 (no. 1): p. 87, March 1979.

9 Gill WB; Schumacher GFB; Bibbo M: Genital and semen abnormalities in adult males two and one-half decades after *in utero* exposure to diethylstilbestrol. Chapter 7 from *Intrauterine Exposure to Diethylstilbestrol in the Human. Proceedings of "Symposium on DES," 1977.* Edited by Arthur L. Herbst, M.D., the American College of Obstetricians and Gynecologists, Chicago, February 1978.

10 Gill WB; Schumacher GFB; Bibbo M; Straus FH; Schoenberg HW: Association of diethylstilbestrol exposure in utero with cryptorchidism, testicular hypoplasia and semen abnormalities. *Journal of Urology,* Vol. 122: p. 36, July 1979.

11 Greene RR; Burrill MW; Ivy AC: Experimental intersexuality. *American Journal of Anatomy,* p. 305, 1940.

12 Guinan P; Bush I; Ray V; Vieth R; Rao R; Bhatti R: The accuracy of the rectal examination in the diagnosis of prostate carcinoma. *New England Journal of Medicine,* Vol. 303 (no. 9): p. 499, August 28, 1980.

13 Henderson BE; Benton B; Cosgrove M; Baptista MA; Aldrich J; Townsend D; Hart W; Mack T: Urogenital tract abnormalities in sons of women treated with diethylstilbestrol. *Pediatrics,* Vol. 58 (no. 4): p. 505, October 1976.

14 Henderson BE; Benton B; Jing J; Yu MC; Pike MC: Risk factors for cancer of the testes in young men. *International Journal of Cancer,* Vol. 23: p. 598, 1979.

15 Hinman F Jr: Unilateral abdominal cryptorchidism. *The Journal of Urology,* Vol. 122: p. 71, July 1979.

16 Kaplan NM: Male pseudohermaphrodism; report of a case with observations on pathogenesis. *New England Journal of Medicine,* Vol. 261 (no. 13): p. 641, September 24, 1959.

17 Kolb FO; Camarg CA: Chapter 18, Endocrine Disorders. From *Current Medical Diagnosis and Treatment,* Lange Medical Publications, Los Altos, California, 1980.

18 Krupp Marcus A: Chapter 15, Genitourinary Tract Tumors of the Testis. From *Current Medical Diagnosis and Treatment.* Edited by Marcus A. Krupp and Milton J. Chaton. Lange Medical Publications, Los Altos, California, 1980.

19 Manber Malcolm M: Diethylstilbestrol. *Medical World News,* p. 44, August 23, 1976.

20 Mills JL; Bongiovanni AM: Effect of prenatal estrogen exposure on male genitalia. *Pediatrics* (supplement), Vol. 62 (no. 6): part 2: p. 1160, December 1978.

21 Ravera J; Pearlman CK; Martin DC: Self-examination of the testes. From a brochure published by Norwich-Eaton Pharmaceuticals, Norwich, New York, April 1976.

22 Rogers BJ; Van Campen H; Ueno M; Lambert H; Bronson R; Hale R: Analysis of human spermatozoal fertilizing ability using zona-free ova. *Fertility and Sterility*, Vol. 32 (no. 6): p. 664, December 1979.

23 Schottenfeld D; Warshauer ME; Sherlock S; Zauber AG; Leder M; Payne R: The epidemiology of testicular cancer in young adults. *American Journal of Epidemiology*, Vol. 112 (no. 2): pp. 232–246, 1980.

24 Scorer CG; Farrington GH: Congenital Anomalies of the Testes, Chapter 44,Volume II, *Campbell's Urology*. Edited by Harrison, Gittes, Perlmutter, Stamey, and Walsh; W. B. Saunders Co., Philadelphia, 1979.

25 Sherins RJ; Howards SS: Male Infertility. Chapter 21, Volume I, *Campbell's Urology*. Edited by Harrison, Gittes, Perlmutter, Stamey, and Walsh; W. B. Saunders Co., Philadelphia, 1979.

26 Sholiton LJ; Srivastava L; Taylor BB: The in vitro and in vivo effects of diethylstilbestrol on testicular synthesis of testosterone. *Steroids*, Vol. 26 (no. 6): pp. 797–806, December 1975.

27 Watson RA; Tang DB: The predictive value of prostatic acid phosphatase as a screening test for prostatic cancer. *New England Journal of Medicine*, Vol. 303 (no. 9): p. 497, August 28, 1980.

Information for this chapter was also obtained from personal interviews with Dr. William Gill (University of Chicago) and Dr. Morton Stenchever (University of Washington).

## CHAPTER 6

1 Bibbo M; Haenszel WM; Wied GL; Hubby M; Herbst AL: A twenty-five year follow-up study of women exposed to diethylstilbestrol during pregnancy. *New England Journal of Medicine*, Vol. 298 (no. 14): p. 763, April 6, 1978.

2 Brian DD; Tilley BC; Labarthe DR; O'Fallon WM; Noller KL; Kurland LT: Breast cancer in DES-exposed mothers. Absence of association. *Mayo Clinic Proceedings*, Vol. 55: pp. 89–93, 1980.

3 Budoff PW: *No More Menstrual Cramps and Other Good News.* Chapter 4, "No More Radical Mastectomies," p. 118, G. P. Putnam's Sons, New York, 1980.

4 Cancer of the Breast: Guidelines for Cancer Related Check-Up. *CA—A Cancer Journal for Clinicians,* published by the American Cancer Society, Vol. 30 (no. 4): pp. 224–229, July/August 1980.

5 Crile G Jr: Management of breast cancer; limited mastectomy. *Delaware Medical Journal,* Vol. 50: pp. 551–556, October 1978.

6 Dowden RV; McCraw JB; Dibbell DG: The breast reconstruction patient and her health insurance carrier. *JAMA,* Vol. 242 (no. 25): p. 2779, December 21, 1979.

7 Fox MA: On the diagnosis and treatment of breast cancer. *JAMA,* Vol. 241 (no. 5): p. 489, February 2, 1979.

8 Gonzalez ER: Vitamin E relieves most cystic breast disease; may alter lipids, hormones (from Medical News column). *JAMA,* Vol. 244 (no. 10): p. 1077, September 5, 1980.

9 Ibid: For others, methylxanthine withdrawal may work.

10 Hoover R; Gray LA Sr; Fraumeni JF Jr: Stilbestrol (diethylstilbestrol) and the risk of ovarian cancer. *The Lancet,* p. 533, September 10, 1977.

11 Hulka BS; Kaufman DG; Fowler WC; Grimson RC; Greenberg BG: Predominance of early endometrial cancers after long-term estrogen use. *JAMA,* Vol. 244 (no. 21): p. 2419, November 28, 1980.

12 Lyle KC: Female breast cancer: distribution, risk factors, and effect of steroid contraception. *Obstetrical and Gynecological Survey,* Vol. 35 (no. 7): p. 413, 1980.

13 Mahoney LJ; Bird BL; Cooke GM: Annual clinical examination: the best available screening test for breast cancer (from the Medical Intelligence column), *New England Journal of Medicine,* Vol. 301 (no. 6): p. 315, August 9, 1979.

14 Matallana R: Expanding role of mammography. *Wisconsin Medical Journal,* Vol. 78: p. 53, August 1979.

15 Medical News: Compromise reached on suggested intervals between Pap tests. *JAMA,* Vol. 244 (no. 13): p. 1411, September 26, 1980.

16 Medical News: New era in treatment of localized breast cancer: Radiation therapy as primary treatment. *JAMA,* Vol. 242 (no. 1): pp. 14–15, July 6, 1979.

17 Montague ED; Guitierrez AE; Barker JL; Tapley N du V; Fletcher GH: Conservation surgery and irradiation for the treatment of favorable breast cancer. *Cancer*, Vol. 43 (no. 3): p. 1058, March 1979.

18 Paffenbarger RS; Elfriede F; Simmons ME; Kampert JB: Cancer risk as related to use of oral contraceptives during fertile years. *Cancer* (supplement), Vol. 39 (no. 4): p. 1820, April 1977.

19 Prosnitz LR: Radiation therapy as initial treatment for breast cancer; is mastectomy necessary? *Connecticut Medical Journal*, Vol. 42 (no. 10): p. 639, October 1978.

20 Segaloff A; Maxfield WS: The synergism between radiation and estrogen in the production of mammary cancer in the rat. *Cancer Research*, Vol. 31: p. 166, February 1971.

21 Shellabarger CJ; McKnight B; Stone JP; Holtzman S: Interaction of dimethylbenzanthracene and diethylstilbestrol on mammary adenocarcinoma formation in female ACE rats. *Cancer Research*, Vol. 40 (no. 6): p. 1808, June 1980.

22 Ultrasound breast examination. From DES Action *Voice*, Vol. 2 (no. 2): p. 8, 1980.

23 Wiggins JP; Rothenbacher H; Wilson LL: Histologic evaluation of the effects of diethylstilbestrol and zeranol on certain lamb tissues. *American Journal of Veterinary Research*, Vol. 41 (no. 4): pp. 487–492, April 1980.

24 Wolfe, Sidney M: Statement to the Food and Drug Administration's Obstetrics and Gynecology Advisory Committee (Evidence of Breast Cancer from DES and Current Prescribing of DES and Other Estrogens), January 30, 1978.

In addition to the above references, information for this chapter was obtained through personal interviews with Dr. Raul Matallana (University of Wisconsin).

## CHAPTER 7

1 Blaska D: Banned DES used at area feedlot: U.S. *The Capital Times* (Madison, Wisconsin), April 10, 1980.

2 Burroughs, Wise: Method of raising beef cattle and sheep and feed rations for use therein. Application to the United States Patent Office for use of DES as growth stimulant in cattle feed, patented June 19, 1956.

3 Burroughs, Wise; Culbertson CC; Cheng E; Hale WH; Nomeyer P: The influence of oral administration of diethylstilbestrol to beef cattle. *Journal of Animal Science,* Vol. 14 (no. 4): p. 1015, November 1955.

4 Burroughs Wise; Culbertson CC; Kastelic J; Cheng E; Hale WH: The effects of trace amounts of diethylstilbestrol in rations of fattening steers. *Science,* Vol. 120 (no. 3106): pp. 266–267, July 9, 1954.

5 Califano, Joseph: press release warning of the dangers of DES issued through the Department of Health, Education, and Welfare. October 4, 1978.

6. Carcinogen used in cattle despite federal ban. *Consumer Reports,* p. 529, September 1980.

7 Feller, William F: Mammography guidelines. DES Action *Voice,* vol. 2 (no. 2): Summer 1980.

8 Griffen, Daniel: personal communication, November 6, 1980. (Mr. Daniel is the executive director of the Iowa State University Research Foundation, Inc., Ames, Iowa).

9 Guarini, Rep. Frank: House of Representatives Bill #6546, introduced to the 96th Congress, 2nd session. (A bill to provide federal financial assistance to states for identifying and examining women exposed to DES; submitted for discussion, but sent back to committee.)

10 Horowitz, Wendy: DES and Government/DES Fed to Cattle. DES Action *Voice,* Summer 1980.

11 Johnson, Anita; Wolfe, Sidney: Letter to Commissioner of the Food and Drug Administration, Dr. Charles Edwards, urging ban on DES as morning-after birth control pill, December 8, 1972.

12 Johnson, Anita; Wolfe, Sidney: Letter to Senator Edward Kennedy urging limitation of DES in animal feed, April 22, 1975.

13 Kennedy, Donald: Modern Medicines: Miracle or Menace? The tenth in a series of 15 articles exploring "The Nation's Health," a program of the University of California, San Diego, and funded by a grant from the National Endowment for the Humanities. Reprinted in the *Wisconsin State Journal,* March 22, 1981.

14 Lanier AP; Noller KL; Decker DG; Elveback LR; Kurland LT: Cancer and stilbestrol; a follow-up of 1,719 persons exposed to estrogens in utero and born 1943–1959. *Mayo Clinic Proceedings,* Vol. 48: p. 793, November 1973.

15 National Cancer Institute: special communication—Information for Physicians on DES, September 17, 1976.

16 Nine out of ten "DES" babies have vaginal adenosis. *Medical World News,* p. 17, November 9, 1973.

17 O'Brien PC; Noller KL; Robboy SJ; Barnes AB; Kaufman RH; Tilley BC; Townsend DE: Vaginal epithelial changes in young women enrolled in the National Cooperative Diethylstilbestrol Adenosis (DESAD) Project. *Obstetrics and Gynecology,* Vol. 53 (no. 3): p. 300, March 1979.

18 Preston R; Cheng E; Story CD; Homeyer P; Pauls J; Burroughs W: The influence of oral administration of diethylstilbestrol upon estrogenic residues in the tissues of beef cattle. *Journal of Animal Science,* Vol. 15 (no. 1): p. 3, February 1956.

19. Richmond, Julius: Physician Advisory; Health Effects of the Pregnancy Use of Diethylstilbestrol. Surgeon-General's advisory sent to physicians across the country, October 4, 1978.

20 Robboy SJ; Kaufman RH; Prat J; Welch WR; Gaffey RT; Scully RE; Richart R; Fenoglio CM; Virata R; Tilley BC: Pathologic findings in young women enrolled in the National Cooperative Diethylstilbestrol Adenosis (DESAD) Project. *Obstetrics and Gynecology,* Vol. 53 (no. 3): p. 309 March 1979.

21 Sestili, Mary Ann: Brief report on the DESAD Project; Genital tract abnormalities and cancer in females exposed in utero to diethylstilbestrol. *Public Health Reports,* September/October 1977.

22 Townsend DE; Hatar P; O'Brien PC: Fertility and outcome of pregnancy in women exposed in utero to diethylstilbestrol. *New England Journal of Medicine,* Vol. 302: pp. 609–613, March 13, 1980.

23 Wolfe, Sidney: statement to FDA Advisory Committee on the Use of Estrogens During Menopause, December 16, 1975.

24 Wolfe, Sidney: Letter to Secretary Joseph Califano about breast cancer in DES mothers, December 12, 1977.

25 Wolfe, Sidney: Evidence of breast cancer from DES and current prescribing of DES and other estrogens. Statement made to the Obstetrics and Gynecology Committee of the FDA, January 30, 1978.

Information for this chapter was also taken from interviews with Dr. Leonard Kurland of the Mayo Clinic, and Dr. Lawrence Ressegnie.

# CHAPTER 8

1 Associated Press: Senator proposes DES bill. *The Independent & Gazette* (California), dateline, Sacramento, California, January 29, 1980.

2 Associated Press: Appeal upheld against Eli Lilly & Co. *The Capital Times* (Madison, Wisconsin), February 25, 1981.

3 Bruck, Connie: Defense lawyers fight over strategy as massive DES battle heats up. *The American Lawyer,* February 1979.

4 The DES cases: a new form of collective liability. Product Liability Trends (published by the Research Group, Inc., Charlottesville, VA 22906), Vol. 4 (no. 5): June 1980.

5 The DES controversy: Part II. Product Liability Trends, Vol. 4 (no. 6): June 1980.

6 *Ferrigno vs. Eli Lilly and Co.* N.J. Super. L, 420, A2d 1305, decided July 2, 1980.

7 Glebatis DM; Janerich DT: A statewide approach to diethylstilbestrol—the New York program. *New England Journal of Medicine,* Vol. 304 (no. 1): p. 47, January 1, 1981.

8 Gorney, Cynthia: DES: The drug, the stricken daughters, and the million-dollar suits. *The Washington Post,* September 7, 1979.

9 Julien, Alfred S; Shainwald, Sybil: Litigation in DES cases. DES Action *Voice,* Vol. 2 (no. 3): Winter 1980.

10 *Mink, Patsy Takemoto et al. vs. University of Chicago et al.* United States District Court, N.D. Illinois, E.D. On motion to dismiss amended complaint October 13, 1978. *Mink v. University of Chicago,* 460 F. Supp. 713 (1978).

11 *Needham, Anne vs. White Laboratories, Inc.* United States Court of Appeals for the Seventh Circuit, No. 80–1579, January 27, 1981. (Pending as of April, 1981).

12 Rout, Lawrence: Product-liability law is in flux as attorneys test a radical doctrine; California Court allows suit citing several producers if maker is unidentified; DES daughters go to court. *The Wall Street Journal,* December 30, 1980.

13 *Sindell, Judith vs. Abbott Laboratories.* L.A. 31063 Supreme Court of California, March 20, 1980 (163 California Reporter 132, 607 Pac 2d 924).

14 Still TW: Battle brews over product liability. *Wisconsin State Journal* (Madison), February 16, 1981.

# CHAPTER 9

1 Associated Press: More don'ts for pregnant mothers. *Wisconsin State Journal,* Section 1: p. 17, September 7, 1980.

2 Associated Press: Morning-sickness drug probed, alleged to cause birth defects. *Wisconsin State Journal,* Section 1: p. 20, September 14, 1980.

3 Barber HRK: *Quick Reference to OB-GYN Procedures,* second edition: pp. 92–93, J. B. Lippincott, Philadelphia, 1979.

4 Barden TP; Peter JB; Merkatz IR: Ritodrine hydrochloride: a betamimetic agent for use in preterm labor. I. Pharmacology, clinical history, administration, side effects and safety. *Obstetrics and Gynecology,* Vol. 56 (no. 1): p. 1, July 1980.

5 Brown SM; Tejani NA: Terbutaline sulfate in the prevention of recurrence of premature labor. *Obstetrics and Gynecology,* Vol. 57: p. 22, January 1981.

6 Food and Drug Administration: Summary basis of approval of New Drug Application 18-280 for ritodrine hydrochloride. (Yutopar™); applicant—Duphar Laboratories, Inc., Columbus, Ohio, and Merrell-National Laboratories, Cincinnati, Ohio.

7 Jacobs MM; Knight AB; Arias F: Maternal pulmonary edema resulting from betamimetic and glucocorticoid therapy. *Obstetrics and Gynecology,* Vol. 56 (no. 1): p. 56, July 1980.

8 Kirkley WH: Fetal survival—what price? *American Journal of Obstetrics and Gynecology,* Vol. 137 (no. 8): p. 873, August 15, 1980.

9 Light, Davin: Bendectin jury awards Orlando family $20,000. *Sentinel Star* (Orlando, Florida), March 22, 1980.

10 Markatz IR; Peter JB; Barden TP: Ritodrine hydrochloride: A betamimetic agent for use in preterm labor. *Obstetrics and Gynecology,* Vol. 56 (no. 1): p. 7, July 1980.

11 Matsunaga E; Shiota K: Threatened abortion, hormone therapy, and malformed embryos. *Obstetrical and Gynecological Survey,* Vol. 35 (no. 8): p. 521, 1980.

12 Oxorn, Harry: *Human Labor and Birth,* fourth edition, Chapter 42, Appleton-Century-Crofts, New York, 1980.

13 Russell, Christine: Mother can control health of newborn. *Wisconsin State Journal* (originally appeared in the *Washington Star*), September 25, 1979.

14 Schenken RS; Hayashi RH; Valenzuela GV; Castillo MS: Treatment of premature labor with beta-sympathomimetics: Results with isoxuprine. *American Journal of Obstetrics and Gynecology,* Vol. 137: p. 773, August 1, 1980.

15 Taber, Ben Zion: *Manual of Gynecologic and Obstetric Emergencies,* pp. 414–415, W. B. Saunders Company, Philadelphia, 1979.

16 Tye KH; Desser KB; Benchimol A: Angina pectoris associated with use of terbutaline for premature labor. Originally appeared in *JAMA,* Vol. 244: p. 692, 1980; abstracted and comments in *Obstetrical and Gynecological Survey,* Vol. 36 (no. 1): p. 14, January 1981.

17 Wilkinson AR; Aynsley-Green A; Mitchell MD: Persistent pulmonary hypertension and abnormal prostaglandin E levels in preterm infants after maternal treatment with naproxen. Originally appeared in *Archives of the Diseases of Childhood,* Vol. 54: p. 942, 1979; abstracted and comments in *Obstetrical and Gynecological Survey,* Vol. 35 (no. 8): p. 507, 1980.

## CHAPTER 10

1 Agnew LRC: Humanism in medicine. *The Lancet,* September 17, 1977.

2 Armitage KJ; Schneiderman LJ; Bass RA: Response of physicians to medical complaints of men and women. *JAMA,* Vol. 24 (no. 20): p. 2186, May 18, 1979.

3 Duttera MJ: The healer's hand. *JAMA,* Vol. 242 (no. 1): p. 41, July 6, 1979.

4 Green LW: Health promotion policy and the placement of responsibility for personal health care. *Family and Community Health (Controversial and Legal Issues),* Vol. 2 (no. 3): p. 51, November 1979.

5 "If you have a complaint about medical care . . . ," brochure published by the State Medical Society of Wisconsin (Madison, Wisconsin), 1979.

6 McCormack Patricia: Male domination blamed for "sickly" women. *Wisconsin State Journal* (Madison), August 26, 1979.

7 Morris LA; Mazis M; Gordon E: A survey of the effects of oral contraceptive patient information. *JAMA,* Vol. 238 (no. 23): p. 2504, December 5, 1977.

8 Osmond H: God and the doctor. *New England Journal of Medicine,* Vol. 302 (no. 10): p. 555, March 6, 1980.

9 Robin ED: Determinism and humanism in modern medicine. *JAMA,* Vol. 240 (no. 21): p. 2273, November 17, 1978.

# Appendix

## DES ACTION NATIONAL OFFICES—

East Coast—DES Action
          Long Island Jewish-Hillside Medical Center
          New Hyde Park, New York 11040
          Telephone: (516) 775-3450

West Coast—DES Action
          1638-B Haight St.
          San Francisco, California 94117
          Telephone: (415) 621-8032

For addresses and telephone numbers of local offices throughout the country, call either national office.

To obtain a copy of the booklet "If You've Thought About Breast Cancer . . . ," by Rose Kushner, call the National Cancer Institute Public Inquiries Office at (301) 496-6631 or the National Cancer Information Services Hotline at the toll-free number, (800) 638-6694.

## NAMES UNDER WHICH DES HAS BEEN MARKETED

Nonsteroidal Estrogens—

| | |
|---|---|
| Benzestrol | Digestil |
| Chlorotrianisene | Domestrol |
| Comestrol | Estilben |
| Cyren A | Estrobene |
| Cyren B | Estrobene DP |
| Delvinal | Estrosyn |
| DES | Fonatol |
| DesPlex | Gynben |
| Dibestil | Gyneben |
| Dienestrol | H-Bestrol |
| Dienoestrol | Hexestrol |
| Diestryl | Hexoestrol |
| Diethylstilbenediol | Menocrin |
| Diethylstilbestrol dipalmitate | Meprane |
| Diethylstilbestrol diphosphate | Mestilbol |
| Diethylstilbestrol dipropionate | Methallenestril |

Microest
Mikarol
Mikarol forti
Milestrol
Monomestrol
Neo-Oestranol I
Neo-Oestranol II
Nulabort
Oestrogenine
Oestromenin
Oestromon
Orestol
Pabestrol D
Palestrol
Restrol
Stilbal
Stilbestrol
Stilbestronate

Stilbetin
Stilbinol
Stilboestroform
Stilboestrol
Stilestrate
Stilooestrol DP
Stilpalmitate
Stilphostrol
Stil-Rol
Stilronate
Stilrone
Stils
Synestrin
Synestrol
Synthoestrin
Tace
Vallestril
Willestrol

Nonsteroidal Estrogen-Androgen Combinations—
Amperone
Di-Erone
Estan
Metystil
Teserene
Tylandril
Tylosterone

Nonsteroidal Estrogen-Progesterone Combination—
Progravidium

Vaginal Cream Suppositories with Nonsteroidal Estrogens—
AVC cream with Dienestrol
Dienestrol cream

For additional information about cancer-related problems or questions, call the National Cancer Information Service from anywhere in the continental United States, or call the Cancer Information Service nearest you. The following numbers are toll-free, except where designated.

National Cancer Information Service: 800/638-6694

Alabama . . . . . . . . . . . . . . . . . . . . . . . . . . . . . . . . . . . . . . . . . 1-800/292-6201
California (to be dialed from area codes 213, 714, and 805 only)
. . . . . . . . . . . . . . . . . . . . . . . . . . . . . . . . . . . . . . . . 1-800/252-9066
   (all other parts of California, call) . . . . . . . . . . . . . . . . . 213/226-2374*
Connecticut . . . . . . . . . . . . . . . . . . . . . . . . . . . . . . . . . . . . . . 1-800/922-0824
Delaware and southern New Jersey (area code 609) . . . . . . . 800/523-3586
District of Columbia (metropolitan area only) . . . . . . . . . . . 202/636-5700*
Florida . . . . . . . . . . . . . . . . . . . . . . . . . . . . . . . . . . . . . . . . . . 1-800/523-3586
   (for Spanish-speaking persons) . . . . . . . . . . . . . . . . . . . 1-800/432-5955
Dade County . . . . . . . . . . . . . . . . . . . . . . . . . . . . . . . . . . . . . . 305/547-6920*
   (for Spanish-speaking persons) . . . . . . . . . . . . . . . . . . . 305/547-6960*
Georgia . . . . . . . . . . . . . . . . . . . . . . . . . . . . . . . . . . . . . . . . . 1-800/327-7332
Hawaii (Oahu only) . . . . . . . . . . . . . . . . . . . . . . . . . . . . . . . . . . . 536-0111*
   (for all other islands) ask operator for Enterprise 6702
Illinois . . . . . . . . . . . . . . . . . . . . . . . . . . . . . . . . . . . . . . . 800/972-0586
   Chicago . . . . . . . . . . . . . . . . . . . . . . . . . . . . . . . . . . . 312/226-2371*
Kentucky . . . . . . . . . . . . . . . . . . . . . . . . . . . . . . . . . . . . . . . 800/432-9321
   (for persons dialing the Kentucky service
   from out-of-state) . . . . . . . . . . . . . . . . . . . . . . . . . . . . . 606/233-6333*
Maine . . . . . . . . . . . . . . . . . . . . . . . . . . . . . . . . . . . . . . . . . . 1-800/225-7034
Maryland . . . . . . . . . . . . . . . . . . . . . . . . . . . . . . . . . . . . . . . . 800/492-1444
Massachusetts . . . . . . . . . . . . . . . . . . . . . . . . . . . . . . . . . . . . 1-800/225-7034
Minnesota . . . . . . . . . . . . . . . . . . . . . . . . . . . . . . . . . . . . . . . 1-800/582-5262
New Hampshire . . . . . . . . . . . . . . . . . . . . . . . . . . . . . . . . . . . 1-800/225-7034
New Jersey (for persons calling from area code 201 only) . . . 800/223-1000
New York State . . . . . . . . . . . . . . . . . . . . . . . . . . . . . . . . . . 1-800/462-7255
   New York City . . . . . . . . . . . . . . . . . . . . . . . . . . . . . . . 212/794-7982*
North Dakota and South Dakota . . . . . . . . . . . . . . . . . . . . . 800/328-5188
North Carolina . . . . . . . . . . . . . . . . . . . . . . . . . . . . . . . . . . . 800/672-0943
Ohio . . . . . . . . . . . . . . . . . . . . . . . . . . . . . . . . . . . . . . . . . . 800/282-6522
Pennsylvania . . . . . . . . . . . . . . . . . . . . . . . . . . . . . . . . . . . . . 800/822-3963
Texas . . . . . . . . . . . . . . . . . . . . . . . . . . . . . . . . . . . . . . . . . 1-800/392-2040
   Houston . . . . . . . . . . . . . . . . . . . . . . . . . . . . . . . . . . . 713/792-3245*
Vermont . . . . . . . . . . . . . . . . . . . . . . . . . . . . . . . . . . . . . . . . 800/225-7034
Washington . . . . . . . . . . . . . . . . . . . . . . . . . . . . . . . . . . . . . 1-800/552-7212
Wisconsin . . . . . . . . . . . . . . . . . . . . . . . . . . . . . . . . . . . . . . 1-800/362-8038

---

*local number; this is a toll call if dialed from outside local area.

# Index